HOW TO MANAGE FAMILY ILLNESS AT HOME

How to Manage

Family Illness at Home

GILL PHARAOH

'An ounce of help is worth a pound of pity.'
Old English proverb

ꓮꓭovvering Books

Copyright © Gill Pharaoh 2004
First published in 2004 by Free Association Books
Revised edition published by Bovvering Books 2013
2A Grange Gardens, Pinner, Middx HA 5 5QE
www.yesiambovvered.com

Distributed by Lightning Source

The right of Gill Pharaoh to be identified as the author of the
work has been asserted herein in accordance with the Copyright,
Designs and Patents Act 1988.

British Library Cataloguing in Publication Data
A catalogue record for this book is available from the British
Library

ISBN 978-0-9562909-1-5

Typeset by Amolibros, Milverton, Somerset
www.amolibros.co.uk
This book production has been managed by Amolibros
Printed and bound by Lightning Source

Contents

Explanation and Introduction

Reviewing this book was a labour of love. In many ways, given her broad experience in a variety of different areas, Gill is uniquely placed to write this sort of book in which she has combined a personal and professional outlook. I think it will appeal broadly both to patients, carers and professionals. In particular, it will be an extremely valuable resource to be turned to by those thrown into the situation of facing terminal illness.

It should also appeal to hospital and community-based professionals as it presents an unusual perspective, bridging patient and carer concerns, but seen through the eyes of an extremely experienced and knowledgeable professional.

In this review I have deliberately avoided areas where I might slightly disagree about emphasis. This book represents a highly personal view, reflecting a unique perspective on a difficult subject. However, it is important to note that Gill has deliberately sought to avoid excessive technical discussion. In particular there are only brief details of drugs or interventions such as catheters, oxygen cylinders or mechanical support including ventilation. I think that this was wise – medical fashions change regularly but this book concerns more permanent issues.

The use of individual case studies is a particularly valuable technique providing the patients are carefully made anonymous. One has to be a little careful however, as some patients and carers have differing views among themselves and with others. It is important not to seem judgemental or pejorative of certain attitudes. Gill treads very carefully and, in her usual tactful manner, avoids these criticisms. On the contrary the use of individual cases does serve to highlight issues in a way that the most detailed scientific medical writing fails to do.

I greatly favour the general tenor of the book with an emphasis on caring at home – we have gradually drifted away from this approach yet the truth is that most patients with terminal illness spend the vast majority of their time, not in hospital or hospice, but at home surrounded by their family. I recognise Gill's point that people change with the sudden and often devastating demands of unexpected severe illness and dependency. This change is reflected in both patient and carer and can place intolerable strain on both parties and the rest of the family, often including children.

The structure and order of the chapters is thoughtful and, like Tony Benn, I greatly appreciate the emphasis on the carer at an early stage and not, as occurs in other books, tagged on as an afterthought.

'Handling death appropriately' is so important. Most people rarely have experience of anyone dying in front of them and, when it is a loved one, the experience can be devastating. Gill copes with this issue in a careful and sensitive manner, which would be of enormous comfort and help to those placed in this position afterwards. There remains an enduring wish among many bereaved to look back and blame themselves for something done or not done. Similarly a sense of anger towards their loved one, themselves or, more commonly, towards the carers or doctors can be the overwhelming emotion experienced. Again, it will be a source of relief to many to realise that they are not unique and that these experiences are in fact relatively common.

There are really so many points raised by this book that I cannot go through them all. In any case I largely agree with Gill's views on management and I greatly applaud the sensitivity and shrewd way that she has been able to illustrate the issues using individual experience but without causing any offence. I would be happy to provide a more detailed review if necessary.

I have not undertaken a detailed critique of all that is being written as this is neither my role nor is it necessary. However, I must emphasise that I have attempted to highlight a few of the reasons why I considered this book to be an extremely valuable contribution to the literature concerning terminal illness for patients, carers and professionals. It is a book that 'needed to be written' and I am delighted that Gill has crafted such an outstanding and valuable contribution.

Robin Howard, Consultant Neurologist, National Hospital for Neurology and Neurosurgery, London May 2004

Foreword by Tony Benn

This sensitive and compassionate book is about palliative care, which concentrates on the patient rather than the illness, and the author has had a long personal experience of work with those who are dying and those who care for them and their families. It is the most moving and useful guide as to what to expect and how to deal with the many problems they face.

It is immensely readable and interesting because it is illustrated with many personal stories and deals with every possible aspect including the emotional needs of the family when they hear of terminal illness, who they should tell and how it should be done, including the responsibility of telling children, how that news is taken and how they may be helped to survive the emotional stress.

It has advice on staying at work for as long as possible and what happens when it is no longer possible to do so, and has a very important chapter on caring for the carers, who are so often overlooked, are under tremendous strain and need respite care themselves, and time to recover from the stress they experience.

We read about the physical needs of those who are ill, how they should deal with medication, and how they can access mechanical aids and appliances, taking into account the problems that are faced by families when mental health may be affected, with an account of the wonderful contribution made by hospices.

One of the most sensitive sections deals with the role of anger by patient and carer, giving advice about depression and isolation, and recognising that many people towards the end argue for euthanasia and even plan suicide.

Inevitably, since the illnesses described lead to death, Gill Pharaoh offers us advice on dying at home or in hospitals, how a funeral can be arranged, and how to deal with bereavement, including advice on what to say and what not to say.

Her last section looks forward to the problems of starting a new life, which is very difficult for those who are left alone, and have to plan for a future without their loved one, even touching on the issue of new relationships that may open up and how to cope with them.

Like many families, I lived through my wife's long illness and tried to provide what care I could when she knew she was dying and was determined to live her life to the full and enjoy every minute of it, arguing that she was not battling against cancer but living happily with it – only regretting that she would not live to see our grandchildren grow up.

She said it was a test of character, and so it was, and I realised that she had taught me how to live and how to die, but how I wish we had had this book to consult during those stressful four years before she was released.

Many books are published about birth, sex, marriage and relationships, and many lifestyle programmes appear on television and personal stories are printed in our newspapers, but we hear very little about death, though it is an experience common to us all.

This is a truly remarkable book; it should be on everyone's shelves, either to consult when needed or to lend to friends who have to cope with the many difficulties we all have when we face the end.

Despite the fact that it is about death Gill Pharaoh gives us hope and brings out the best in human nature, which sometimes happens when people are faced with a real crisis, and find themselves struggling with problems that are unknown until they arise, and in circumstances that are beyond their direct control.

Tony Benn, 4th April 2004

Author's Note

I would like to thank the following people for the part they have played in finally getting this book on the shelf.

First of all my family, Caron and Mark, who from a very young age encouraged and supported me in my career changes, and from great distances, still do. Now joined by Jill and grandson Reuben.

And thank you to John, my long-time partner, who has given a lot of his valuable time to advise, instruct, criticise, and support me for the last twenty years (skills not always appreciated at the time!). He has also proved to be an excellent secretary!

Many thanks to Robin Howard, consultant neurologist at the National Neurological Hospital, Queen Square, for his thoughtful and helpful review of this book, and to Tony Benn, for his enthusiastic and generous foreword.

I owe a great deal to Philippa Gale, my oldest friend, and to Yvonne Thomas, for their patience and skill in reading and re-reading this manuscript and being truthful in their comments and generous with their time.

Most of all, I remember the many people who influenced me over the years; some were my co-workers, specialists in their field, but most were those sick people and their families, with whom I became very close for a short and sad time, and from whom I learned so much.

And finally, I would like to put on record my special thanks to Jane Tatam from Amolibros for her generous support, advice and guidance throughout the publication of this book, and my previous book *Careers in Caring*.

Introduction

Why this book?

Every day, hundreds of people make an unexpected transition from housewife, mother, friend, lover, son, daughter, to 'carer'. They usually have little warning, no real chance of refusing, and very little idea of what is expected of them. These people may be family members, neighbours, men or women, old people and children as young as nine years old, and sometimes even younger.

What is a carer? Is this a new role? Why haven't we noticed this happening in our communities in the past?

Not so long ago there was time to recover from a hospital experience while the patient was still in hospital. Hospital admissions were planned to a large extent, and people were admitted on the expected date, usually the day before the operation or treatment. People were in hospital for long enough after their surgery to be able to sit around the ward, to help out less able patients, and gradually become a little stronger. Often before returning home they were also offered a week or two in a convalescent home or a cottage hospital. Generally the district nurse followed through the care once they were back home, to make sure they were managing well, and to reassure and support them as they returned to full health. When medical staff talked about community care, that was what they meant. And most important of all, once at home, many of the patients were within reach of family, and had neighbours whom they knew well who had the time to pop in and out, and help out on a regular basis. The result was that the patient had time to regain their confidence, which often takes quite a knock if the illness is unexpected.

The tendency today is for people to spend as short a time as possible in hospital. In theory, this suits the average person very well indeed, since most people do not particularly enjoy their stay in hospital, and prefer the familiarity of their own home. Their admission is often in doubt until the last minute because of shortage of beds, so they are less able to make definite plans for their return home. For someone in pain, or anxious about their health, this uncertainty about the dates increases their anxiety.

Modern, improved techniques in surgery and anaesthetics, and greater understanding about the process of healing, mean less trauma, and less time in bed for the patient, who is encouraged to start moving as soon as possible. This is better for the patients physically, but is also often rather traumatic as well, giving them no time to settle in and to get to know the staff caring for them. And if they have fairly major treatment they have no time to recover their self-confidence following the hospital experience.

Changes in the way the National Health Service is managed mean that 'care in the community' is now normally the preferred option of hospital staff, and community staff. Hospital care is expensive, and beds must be given the maximum use. Hospitals are more specialised, there is often a shortage of nurses and doctors as well as technicians in all areas, porters and all the other staff required to support a stay in hospital. Also hospitals resort to using agency staff, so the continuity is lacking for both staff and patient.

For all these reasons the patient is sent home as soon as is possible, and the bed used again for someone who can be easily identified as more in need of a bed. So people are leaving hospital when they are still physically weak and still in need of nursing care. As a result 'care in the community' has come to mean a much more intensive and broad-ranging service, covering *all* aspects of illness, including many treatments traditionally given while in hospital, up to and including the death of a person. If it is possible to continue a treatment at home, then the patient will be discharged.

Unfortunately as all these changes were in process, the smaller hospitals that often gave good convalescent care, and also dealt with minor illnesses and operations, were being closed. Experienced staff who did not want to work in high-pressure intensive units left the profession and were not replaced.

Working in the community, in the homes of sick and often frightened people, is a skill that district nurses and healthcare workers are not necessarily born with, but that takes time and experience to develop. Even if the desire to care is instinctive, the expertise is not. It is a learned skill. It takes time and strong motivation, which many carers do not necessarily have.

District nurses and GPs are trying to deal with huge numbers of patients and a massive increase in paperwork and record keeping. Many district nurses now have a caseload of more than ninety sick people on their books, compared with thirty or so only thirty years ago. They cannot make the time to listen and support in the way they would choose to do. They no longer forge the same strong bonds with members of their local community, because they do not know them in the same way. Record-keeping regulations mean that the district nurses of today have very strict time limits imposed on them, which do not allow for the quick informal visit that, in the past, often prevented problems developing, or at the very least anticipated and identified them earlier.

In the main, people suddenly projected into the new role of carer do a remarkable job. Even with a great deal of help it is still a sad and painful path to have to take. If they get only minimal support, the carers pay a huge personal price, and this is often a source of concern to the person who is ill and to the relatives. It also protracts the effect of the illness and often leads to mental and physical illness after it is all over. At the very least, it makes coping with bereavement all the more difficult.

However, there is another side to the situation. If someone can be cared for at home with support and help from the right people, the whole experience can be valuable and memorable, and, even when it ends with the death of a loved one, can be experienced as a source of satisfaction and comfort to everyone concerned.

This book tries to give some ideas on how to manage some of the situations that may be met by the carer, and the person for whom they are caring. It is written for both carer and 'patient', not as a set instruction manual, but as a book to dip into when necessary. It is not about controlling a situation, but about making situations easier, if possible, and at the very least becoming aware of potential difficulties.

Most of the ideas and suggestions written here come from the experiences of ordinary people, who were projected into becoming carers or patients, and learned for themselves ways to make the situation more bearable. Much of what is written here is anecdotal. The characters have been disguised, but these are real people, who dealt with situations they had never expected, or planned for.

When the expression 'terminal illness' has been used, the words conjure up for people an immediate, painful and terrifying death. This makes the whole experience more horrifying for all concerned. It is important to understand the facts. The facts are different. *It is rare that death is immediate, and with good care and support it does not have to be either painful or terrifying. It is a natural process, like birth, with moments of acute sadness, and moments of deep joy.*

What is good care? All the surveys of hospital care indicate that whether or not people can identify good standards of clinical care when they see them, very many sick people and their families do not *feel* that they are getting the care they need. When people describe hospital experiences it is rare that someone says they had a most wonderful machine to X-ray them. They speak of the personal kindness and expertise, the compassion, the nice bath they were given, the one who washed their hair for them, or made them a drink in time of great stress. If the illness progresses, many patients and their families find that they are obsessed by the memories of the quality of the care they received initially. It is very hard for them to put these memories behind them. All too often the care given at home by the 'amateur' carer far surpasses that received in the hospital unit.

Problems of long-term care are similar, and all too often the expected short illness can become long term. By the time this happens, the carer and family are exhausted and stressed, and the patients may feel they are a burden, and no one is able to appreciate the extra time they once prayed for.

Being aware of problems that may occur does not remove the problem, but can often make it more understandable, and therefore more manageable. Long-term illness has several aspects, and may be complicated by dementia (due to further disease like Alzheimer's disease), confusion due to medication or weakness, or chronic depression.

Children can become very difficult when there is a sick person in the home for a long time, and may then experience feelings of guilt and remorse for years afterwards. It is quite common for younger children to feel responsible in some way for the onset of illness, so anticipating and recognising feelings at an early stage can reduce the tension considerably, and lessen some of the after effects.

Euthanasia and suicide are sometimes suggested, in the media, as the alternative to dying as a natural result of a serious illness. People who are dying often do ask for this kind of help. This has also been discussed.

What is the correct procedure following a death at home? Although most people say they would prefer to die at home, only about thirty per cent actually do so, and the prospect of such a death often fills the carers and the family with great apprehension. Many professionals have no experience of someone dying at home, because they have never been there when it happens. Few nurses have the experience of being at a bedside when a person dies in their own bed. It is usually the carer who has to decide what to do.

Some things are very clear: they know they have certain legal obligations. The questions that have not been asked, and therefore are not answered are: Who do you call at the moment of death? Your own doctor, or do you dial 999? Are you supposed to try and resuscitate? Do you do anything to the body? What do you do if children are there? What are you *supposed* to do? What is the *right* thing to do?

People rarely ask these questions in case they appear to be wishing death to occur. Professionals rarely offer the information for fear of upsetting the family. But for many people, this is a question that remains uppermost in their minds for much of the time. And deep regrets after a death can affect the whole course of the bereavement process.

There is also a look at bereavement: what is regarded as 'normal', and what strategies might help a little. Waiting for someone to die affects a wide circle of people, friends as well as family, and there are other losses, which are experienced later, which may not be anticipated initially. There is no right or wrong way to cope, but sometimes hearing how other people have managed can help to clarify feelings.

The reaction of children is often remembered only as an afterthought, or if the child shows signs of distress. Children often cover their feelings to accommodate the adults around them. It is not easy to support them without dictating their responses.

There are also less acceptable emotions, for example when there has been dislike or resentment in the relationship that has been unresolved at the death.

This book does not claim to supply the answers to many questions, but tries to provide enough information to help you find the answers that are right for you.

Chapter One

Receiving the Diagnosis

For many people, the diagnosis of cancer or some other frightening disease comes only after a period of anxiety, fear, and apprehension that may have lasted for months or weeks. Most people have little accurate medical knowledge. Yet with every illness there are myths and gossip, interspersed with truth. When the diagnosis means that someone may well be going to die at some time, and if the disease is cancer, the myths increase in number.

Sitting for long periods in an outpatient clinic watching other people, who appear to be just as ill, or even worse, is not reassuring. Imagination runs riot in a busy outpatients department, particularly a specialist one, where an onlooker almost seems able to observe and chart the progress of an illness. *Symptoms and disease vary with each individual.* It is hard to remember this when faced with a clinic full of people with cancer, or some neurological disease, that holds a threat of early death.

The way a diagnosis is given can make a lot of difference. Doctors are no different from other people, though we usually expect them to be somehow more sensitive. However good their training, they are still very individual people. Some are sensitive about the way they give a diagnosis, and others are not. Some are skilled communicators, and others are more detached, and less comfortable with a face-to-face meeting. Some are sensitive, and others deliver the blunt facts in an almost triumphant way.

People also vary in the way they hear explanations from a doctor. Reactions depend on many factors: how long have they been waiting and undergoing tests? How ill do they feel? It is hard to accept any kind of diagnosis if someone is feeling perfectly well. What kind of personal history do they have?

When they hear the diagnosis, whether it comes as a shock or is half expected, the first question very often is, 'Am I going to die?' and then 'How long have I got?' It is instinctive, because it is the thought uppermost in their minds, and yet for many people it is the last piece of information they really want to hear. Often the reply is very vague: perhaps a doctor will say something like 'From one to five years.' An optimistic person may hear the five louder than the one and feel somewhat reassured. Someone with foreboding and fear may hear only 'one year' and feel they are sitting in death row.

It is easy for people who have not experienced this situation to dismiss the question with platitudes. Pam, when told by her doctor that she could just as easily walk under a bus tomorrow, replied indignantly:

'I am far too careful when I cross the road!'

She was able to laugh at him, but that kind of comment does not help most people at all.

However good or bad a consultant may be at giving a diagnosis, the fact is that few specialists can predict the time of death. The best they can say is that they cannot cure the illness, and try to make a guess, based on the experience of similar patients. To remove all hope from a person may stop them trying to live with an illness, and that makes it hard for everyone. Equally, to urge someone to 'fight the disease' is hardly helpful. Fighting implies physical action of some sort. And what are the feelings of all concerned if the disease does not 'give in'? Does it mean that someone has not fought hard enough? If so, what else could they have done? And with what weapons?

The return of the illness implies massive failure.

This does not mean that a good mental attitude does not have an effect on the course of the disease or illness. Planning ahead with realism and optimism is the middle road, and helps to keep an even balance emotionally, and reduce some of the stress.

With current treatment, and increased knowledge of palliative care, many illnesses can be managed at home, for far longer periods than we used to imagine. However, if, initially, someone has been clumsily treated by their consultant, the anger and hurt at receiving insensitive treatment at such a traumatic time can lead to a lack of confidence in the specialists, and a feeling of helplessness in the face of overwhelming disaster. It makes a great difference to the way someone feels if they can trust in, and communicate with the person who is managing their illness.

Responding to the Diagnosis

Liz was a very successful businesswoman. She had built up a company, and was still working full time when she suspected she had a health problem. Having never been ill, she found the whole experience shocking. She felt very undermined by the impersonal feel of the brand-new hospital; she hated the way she had to wait around half dressed, she found it very hard to feel so out of control of the situation. She had made it quite plain that she needed to know exactly what her situation was, since a lot of people depended on her for their jobs. However, throughout her tests she was told very little, in spite of her questions. On her last appointment her consultant gave her a final examination, then stood opposite her as she sat on the couch in her white cotton X-ray gown, unfastened at the back, feeling very exposed. He said she had an advanced ovarian cancer and would not live to see Christmas, but might see the summer out. He waited a few moments and when, in her shocked state, she said nothing, he told her there was no curative treatment he could sensibly offer, but that he would review her case on a regular basis, and left.

Liz found that she was unable to forget the experience. She brooded for weeks, wishing she had been able to say something. She talked non-stop about her anger; she talked about changing consultants and going to a private hospital; she wanted to cancel all further appointments. She did none of these things, but continued to wake, crying, in the night, as she relived her experience. Finally she sat down and wrote the consultant a letter, in which she said that the unpleasant experience of being diagnosed with cancer was made ten times worse by the way she was told her diagnosis. She was very calm and not at all abusive, but she said that she dreaded her next appointment, and feared what might be said to her if she returned. She wondered if she could be referred to a more sympathetic specialist. Then she sent it to her consultant. She had decided that if she did not receive a sympathetic response she would copy the letter to the hospital manager, but she had no need to take it any further. Her consultant wrote back immediately to say he was very sorry indeed, and to thank her for drawing his attention to her distress. He appreciated he had been very unkind, and would like to see her again, and start the relationship on a different footing.

Her next appointment was totally different. He treated her with respect and understanding, and gave her plenty of opportunity to say how she felt. Her treatment thereafter was excellent. Most important of all, she felt more in control, and was able to put her anger behind her, and put all her energy into managing her affairs and looking after her health.

When later she decided to look for some complementary therapies to go with her palliative treatment, the same consultant was very supportive. And she was well enough to enjoy Christmas, and two summers in spite of his prognosis.

Some people will be too frightened, and in awe of the doctors, to attempt such an approach, fearing that they will not receive such good treatment if they are identified as 'difficult patients'. Many people also fear telling the specialists that they are also using other therapies in the way they manage their illness. But for anyone to nurse anger and sadness is very unhealthy, and it is better to be honest, as many doctors are simply unaware of the kind of anguish they cause. For the patient to tell them has more impact than comments from a dozen allied professionals. There have always been conflicting views on complementary therapies, but since they are unlikely to do harm, and are often enjoyable to the recipient, many specialists will neither reject them nor encourage their use.

If, immediately after receiving the diagnosis, the question of how long has been asked and the answer given, then the best thing to do is to plan for the worst scenario, with all the dreaded complications, and then expect the opposite. This advice is easy to give, but it is a fact that often when plans have been made, and everything is settled, there is a feeling of completion and life can be taken a day at a time.

In the course of an illness it is usual for people to feel as good emotionally as they do physically. In other words, a person who has few, or no unpleasant symptoms will feel optimistic and cheerful. Fear makes pain or discomfort much worse.

A Closer Look at the First Reaction to the Diagnosis

The first reaction to the diagnosis is like a bomb exploding in a very small space, and the resulting chaos takes a long time to settle down. Emotions vary from disbelief, to anger, to tears, to despair, and it feels as if life is over already, and nothing will ever be the same again. It feels like a sentence, which affects everyone who is close to the person at the centre. It takes a while to register the implications, and very often there is a longing to identify a cause, something to blame: cigarettes, lifestyle, family history, medical care, stress, neglect, whether their own or by their doctor – in fact anything to give a reason for such disaster. It takes time to accept that awful things can happen to nice people and, while it is hard not to ask why it is important to look for ways to meet the challenge ahead.

So at the beginning, it is wise to sit it out, and wait for the emotional dust to settle. Sometimes people, the patient or the partner, feel they do not want to tell the news to anyone, even close family. Sometimes a couple cannot agree on which action to take. And both can become trapped within these strong emotions, and become deadlocked and unable to move on.

It is fine to say nothing for a short period, but silence and denial deprives everyone of getting the support they need, and may continue to need. Denial also avoids the opportunity to make plans that enable every person involved to make the most of the time they have.

It also deprives close friends or family of the *chance* of giving support. Since it is hard to pretend that all is well when patently it is not, the deception involves everyone in small lies at first, gradually developing into bigger lies, which become difficult to unravel. The progress of the disease is usually inevitable, so eventually the truth will out, and it may take some time to rebuild the trust and respect that has been lost, time that may not be available.

To be given a distressing diagnosis at any time is hard. When it is unexpected and the person concerned feels and looks relatively well, it is understandable if he or she decides to go back to work and say absolutely nothing, or else tell everyone all the details, and then regret it later. If it is possible to have a few days at home, or with the family, to absorb the information and come to some understanding of the situation, then it is easier to make a thoughtful response, and inform only the people who will understand and give their support.

When Intimacy is Affected by the Diagnosis

As we said, sometimes the immediate response to the diagnosis is withdrawal from family and friends, who could be supportive if they were given the chance. Sadly, it is often the partner of the patient who is the first person who feels the rejection. It is not uncommon for the sex life of a couple to be almost immediately affected by the diagnosis, or later on, following surgery or radiation, and this can be a deeply painful response for the partner. A man may no longer be able to sustain an erection, and yet still feel a desire for his partner. Loving touching, stroking and explaining can go a long way to helping them both find solutions that satisfy and express their feelings.

A woman may feel she has become ugly, and unattractive, following surgery or radiation, and may also completely lose any desire for sex. Many people feel they smell, if not unpleasant, at least strange, when they are having treatment. Some relationships are not passionate, and so this may not appear as a problem initially. But if a couple have had a loving and sexually active partnership, losing the physical loving is a very painful part of the illness.

From the start this is something to be discussed and explained. Silence is not the best way to react. Of course, there are a few people who feel less attracted to a damaged body, and find it hard to respond to an invitation to make love, even when they have enjoyed a passionate relationship previously. However, more frequently, it is the fear of causing pain that restrains them, and the partner who is well may need a lot of reassuring. Rarely nowadays is there the fear of catching cancer, or other serious illness, which was often mentioned years ago, when our knowledge was poor, and doctors were less inclined to give information.

If the subject is ignored by the couple, it can only become more painful, if not to both people, then most certainly to one of them. The very best way is to talk together, and work out a solution. Or at least, find a counsellor with whom to discuss the subject, without embarrassment.

Sometimes in the immediate aftermath of the diagnosis, anti-depressants and similar medication are suggested. This is an individual decision of course, and should be discussed with the doctor as often a short course of anti-depressants can help. Although homeopathic remedies are controversial and considered not proven, they have been in use for many years, and sometimes a simple herbal treatment like Bach Flowers Rescue Remedy can alleviate the occasional panic attack, while someone adapts to the news. Many people use a homeopathic remedy to help to banish the kind of thoughts that cause people to lie awake at night worrying. It is very worthwhile asking for advice from a homeopath, and if the remedy does not help, at least it has no unwanted side effects, and is not addictive.

The Fear of Inherited Disease

There is often the question of where does this come from? Who is to blame? Perhaps there have been several deaths in the family of similar causes. The thought of handing such a legacy on to one's children is hard to accept, and is one of the most often voiced anxieties associated with a malignant disease. Some families will comment on an apparent family history, showing a tendency to develop certain illnesses like lung disease or strokes, but this is not the same as an inherited disease, and can often be explained. Few people have an in-depth knowledge of their family illness, and ignorance and imagination increase fear, especially when cancer is mentioned. This needs to be addressed as soon as possible. Of course some diseases are inherited, but very few. The risk is usually not absolute, and learning the facts is always less frightening than the imagined possibilities.

Most specialist cancer or neurological units have experts who can clarify the risk in specific illness, and are glad to speak to anxious relatives. Many of them are pleased to add to their own knowledge by recording family histories. Sometimes this can help the family too, as they feel they are helping to understand and perhaps one day eliminate the disease. The questions have to come from the family, and some members may resist any attempt to discuss the possibility. It has to be a personal choice made without pressure. It is easy to find out where these specialists are from the consultant, or the nurse, or by asking to see a geneticist.

There are many ways of getting information about illness, disease and treatment. Some sources for help are at the end of this book.

Many diseases have a charity specifically formed to help people understand the problems. Usually these are very helpful and well worth using. Often the initial response on diagnosis is to resist the label of something so frightening, but access to reliable information is much more reassuring than trying to deal with a mass of myth and misconception. What we are capable of imagining in the middle of a sleepless night can be far more terrifying than the facts.

The internet gives a great deal of information about many subjects. It is often the first port of call for anyone wanting information in a hurry. It is well to remember that much of the medical information on the internet has not been proven, and is really very subjective, being one person's experience and perception. It is easy to have unrealistic hopes about miracle cures, so while using the source it's wiser to retain a core of scepticism.

Chapter Two

Whom to Tell?

Sometimes a family will try to keep the truth from the person who is ill. This is a common situation with people who have cancer, and may be because of the still limited knowledge about the disease. Many people still believe that cancer means instant and very painful death, or prolonged and very painful death, and so a sick person will collude with the family in the hope that this is not really happening after all.

If someone has always preferred not to know what is happening, this may be effective for a while. But most people know that they are not getting better, because they feel weaker, or because of the attention they receive from everyone around them. Not to mention the unaccustomed doctors and specialists who seem to find them interesting.

Most people know when they are being deceived, and they are aware of emotional undercurrents and whispered conversations going on around them. They may feel a sense of doom, or they may think they are going mad, because everyone says how well they are doing, and yet they feel so ill, or lethargic. Afraid to ask the straight question they will say, 'Am I getting better?' and get an easy reassuring, 'Of course you are' in reply. There is no need to be blunt to the point of cruelty, but if the reply is focussed on *them* and around their perception of how things are, it gives them space to consider how they are really feeling, and permission to question what they have been told. For example 'How do *you* feel you are getting on?' or 'Are you especially worried about something?' or 'Do you have questions that need answering?'

The person who is ill is at the centre of the situation, and how he or she feels is the crux of the matter. Simply supporting them while they come to terms with the diagnosis is the most helpful way to respond. The easy reassurance 'Of course you are getting better, doctors have made a mistake/read the wrong notes/muddled the results with someone else' can only eventually increase the anxiety, and the suspicion they are being lied to.

This does not mean hammering in the truth in a brutal way. It is very common for people to think they have been given the wrong diagnosis and to ask for it to be reassessed and reviewed. They need time to question what is happening. If someone says 'I am getting better every day' or even 'I am getting more and more ill' the only thing to do is to acknowledge those feelings. 'I'm glad because you are the one who knows best of all how you feel.'

Simply accepting how they feel is an important part of supporting them.

Max was forty-five years old and diagnosed with a very rapid type of lung cancer, with a prognosis of about twelve to eighteen months. He was an active and practical man, with a physically demanding job. He was a very keen gardener and DIY expert, always busy with a project at home when he was not working. His wife Phyllis refused to allow the doctors to tell him he had cancer, so there was no starting point for questions. She said he had never wanted to hear bad news, and that this would devastate him, and he would give up immediately. The three adult children were divided in their opinions, but since they all lived away from home with their own families, they went along with her decision. As he became weaker he became quieter and more withdrawn, only watching television and talking very little. Phyllis was calm and remote in company, and wept copious tears whenever she was alone.

Max had a bath twice weekly from a bath attendant who was a mature and calmly efficient lady. One day she said to him, 'You seem really low today. Is there anything you are worried about?' Lying in the warm water, feeling relaxed and comfortable, he suddenly told her he was worried that he was going mad. He had lost so much weight, and he felt so weak the slightest effort left him exhausted. He was completely unable to do any of his usual activities. No one seemed at all surprised by his weakness, and he was either going mad or they were hiding something from him. He had initially suspected that he might have cancer, but the lack of the kind of pain he expected, and the absolute denials of his wife, convinced him otherwise. Now he suspected things were being kept from him.

This, he said, had always been the case with his parents, and he had hoped his marriage would be different. However it was a difficult pattern to break, and throughout the marriage he and Phyllis had kept any bad news from each other, as far as was possible. Now he suspected he had cancer or something worse, and he could not discuss it with her in case she didn't know, and he could not bear to hurt her. Or perhaps she knew, and could not cope with the truth. He even wondered if he had AIDS as the grandchildren no longer called – they waved from the car sometimes, but never came in to see him. He felt he had nothing he could say to them, but he missed playing with them as he used to. All the questions ran around in his brain all day, and half the night. He just wished he were dead and out of it all.

The bath lady persuaded him to allow her to sound out Phyllis without pressurising her, and he reluctantly agreed. As she left him warm and tucked up in bed, she went downstairs to find Phyllis weeping silently as she did the dusting. She gently told her what Max had said. Phyllis immediately ran to talk to him.

The barrier was broken, and for the last few weeks of his life his depression lifted. He was very sad, and there were many tears shed, but he was able to tell the family how much he loved them. How proud he was of them. How good a partner he felt he had always had in Phyllis. The air was cleared in so many small ways. His pain and discomfort lessened with the drop in his anxiety levels. His children were able to be themselves with him. His son was open and able to talk about anything, while his daughters were less so, but they were all aware of the situation now, and there was a relaxation of pressure in this new understanding. His smallest grandson asked him if he was going a long way away and if so, could he please phone him? Max said he could not phone so far, but that he would always be thinking of them, and they must not forget how much he loved them all. The little boy duly reported to his mother that he and his granddad had sorted it all out, and she must not worry. They were all able to laugh at that. He died very peacefully, having said all he wanted to say to his family and his friends, and having heard all that they wanted to say to him. Phyllis said afterwards that she had been afraid that she would never be able to stop crying, but that somehow the weight of pain in her chest had been lifted, and she felt at peace.

David and Joan were a very different couple. They were quiet and introspective, the personification of the small cul-de-sac in which they had lived for fifteen years, where they found it hard to be intimate with friends and neighbours, though they were the first to offer help to anyone else. When the news of Joan's illness became general people approached their daughter Pippa for advice about how to help. Knowing how reserved her parents were, Pippa felt that practical, unobtrusive help would be the most appreciated.

She made a list of things to do, and while the two of them stayed quietly in their home, neighbours and friends delivered meals, did the washing and ironing and mowed the grass. Each task was a small job in itself, but hard to organise, when someone is trying to make sense of such disaster. Although friends saw themselves as giving only practical help to the couple and to Pippa, this was also experienced as emotional support. As a result of the help given, the whole neighbourhood drew closer together.

For many people, this amount of assistance may not be possible, or even welcome. Offers of help are often rejected by the recipient, in a bid to be strong and independent, not realising that anything that eases the stress on the family can only be a blessing. Of course, some help is not welcome. It can be an intrusion to have a deluge of callers at such a time, unless they can be unobtrusive and undemanding. Not many people have someone like Pippa to filter visitors, and allocate jobs.

Making Changes

No decisions have to be made immediately. Life-changing decisions need a lot of careful thought and discussion. Sometimes there is a desire to move house, to be nearer the family, to find a place that is easier to manage should the patient become disabled. These are changes that are not likely to happen overnight. Sometimes there will not be time to make a major change like a house move. Besides, leaving a home behind with all the good memories as well as the sad ones, not to mention the problems of finding a new house, can add to the trauma, and delay the process of acceptance and adaptation.

The desire to move away can also be a longing to leave all this illness behind in the excitement of a new house, or to return to a place with happy earlier memories.

It is better to gather as much information as possible before rushing into decisions that are life changing, and will be difficult or impossible to reverse.

Similarly, a partner often feels they should stop work immediately and prepare to stay at home to look after the ill person. This may be necessary at some time, but usually it is possible to keep a job, especially if it provides more than just financial help, and is a source of help and support to the family. One massive life change at a time is enough to manage. It is a good decision to make *no* decisions about anything, other than what to have for lunch, for at least a few weeks. Talk things over with family or friends, but make no definite plans at all. Accept help. Most people want to help, and are glad to be given suggestions as to what to do.

Talking to Someone

It always helps to have someone to confide in. Sometimes couples provide their own support for each other. Even so, they may need to talk as well to someone outside, who is not so personally affected. It can be hard to find the right person, and even very close friends may not be able to give the responses needed. Most people do not want advice. They want to keep repeating their view of what is happening, and the options open to them, because by constant repetition they are able to absorb the information they have been given, and make their own decision.

When looking for someone to talk to, it is useful to consider a few points about the kind of person who will help. If a friend has repeated confidences regarding other friends, whether mutual or not, then the chances are that they are not safe with confidences, even if they appear very sympathetic. Likewise people who talk a great deal about their own recent or distant loss are often still too wrapped up in their own grief to be able to help you try to make sense of your tragedy. Often relevant charities or support groups have appointed visitors to help and befriend people who are in the throes of the illness.

This all sounds rather calculating. But in other circumstances we would call such forethought, planning. It is a fact that we spend more time planning a two-week holiday than planning our own last few months or years on earth. Many people have no warning that they may die, and they do not have the opportunity to make any plans. For those who do have some warning, why not try to make the experience as rich and fulfilling as possible? This ensures that the experience and the memories are rewarding as well as sad, for the ones left behind.

People who have a strong religious belief and go to a church, or similar meeting place, may find a lot of support in that community. However, this does not apply to so many people nowadays, and they may find that they resent it when visitors push their beliefs onto the family. No one needs to tolerate pressure at such a time, and however well meaning the offers may be it is quite acceptable to refuse to be pressured.

In fact this is the time to be completely selfish and accept only what is helpful and supportive and reject firmly any 'help' that does not feel welcome and comfortable. If a 'Pippa' is available and can be trusted, he or she can be a great asset. If not, then the people at the centre of the situation must take control of this very important time in their lives.

Chapter Three

The Services of the Hospice and Palliative Care Team

The hospice role is still often misunderstood. Many people are very apprehensive about making contact with the local hospice, as it feels to them as if they are applying to die. Also, there is the suspicion that Macmillan nurses, or the palliative care team, will make people talk about dying, or force knowledge on families and patients who are not ready to think too hard about the future for the time being.

There is the common myth that a hospice exists for people on the point of death. In fact hospice is not so much a building, as a service for people with life-threatening illness. The best hospice services provide support, symptom control and advice *throughout* an illness, and the majority of people who come within the hospice service do not die in the hospice, but choose to remain at home. Many people will be inpatients several times, over many months, for respite care and assessment. Some will go once for assessment, and some never become inpatients at all. And some will go there to die. Many people also receive hospice care in nursing homes, and hospitals. A hospice should be a flexible option, to meet the individual needs of the patient, and the family. Indeed nowadays some hospices offer a home nursing service for people who never want to be admitted at all.

Macmillan nurses, and other community palliative care teams, should offer emotional support, and the opportunity to talk things over, *if* that is what the patient wants. They will also be able to support the families and friends if the person wants to die at home. For many families, the idea of someone dying at home is very frightening, and although they may agree with the concept, they are scared of how they will manage when the time comes. And yet not so long ago this was the normal place for death to occur. And for most people it is still where they hope to be, if it is possible and if the support is there.

As well as emotional support the Macmillan or palliative care team will also be able to monitor and advise on symptom control. The patient and family do not have to accept any form of pressure, if they are not happy with what is on offer, for whatever reason.

Palliative care offers the holistic care of the patient together with the treatment of the symptoms of a disease, at a time when the hope of a cure has passed. Therefore the intention is not to cure, but to keep the patient comfortable, and free from unpleasant or uncomfortable physical symptoms, as well as supporting them through the emotional and spiritual distress they may be experiencing. In the early days, many hospices were only able to offer this care to people with cancer, but it was soon realised that many illnesses that are not immediately going to cause death can cause a great deal of misery, which might make someone wish to die. Some services took time to expand to include other diagnoses, because the initial funding was specifically for the person with cancer. Now, many palliative care teams use their skills to make life comfortable for people who cannot be cured of illness or disease.

The way to find out the extent of your local services is to

make contact, see if you can visit yourself, or ask someone to visit for you, and ask lots of questions!

Facts About Medication

There is also a myth that hospices put people to sleep to spare them pain, and even kill them painlessly. This is also quite untrue, as well as being against the law, and it would be hard, if not impossible, to staff a place with such a bleak approach to illness!

The fact is that any medication has some side effects, apart from the main aim of relieving a symptom. For example, the leaflet that comes with morphine may warn about taking it if there are breathing problems involved. This may be true for a well person, but if someone has severe breathing difficulties, and is terribly frightened, the effect of the drug on their breathing is going to be minimal, compared with the improvement that a reduction in symptoms will have. If it is prescribed, it may be because the doctor believes that by reducing the fear and stress on someone struggling for breath, the breathlessness can be helped. The word morphine is apt to cause anxiety and conjures up visions of addiction. Again the best approach is to ask questions, and more questions (never be afraid of appearing foolish!), or else decide the specialists know their job, and are trying to help you, and put your trust in them, and let them get on with it.

Any comment on medication given in this book is very general. The main aim is to encourage you and your family to keep informed about the reasons for whatever actions are being taken.

For some people the services and support of a hospice can be very valuable.

Within the hospice services there are people who can talk through the diagnosis, and explain the kind of support that is on offer. Looking round and talking about options is not a commitment, but may serve to open up new possibilities.

When is the Best Time to Make Contact?

It is wise to make early contact with a hospice, as part of the process of planning for whatever lies ahead. Also hospices vary considerably in the way they operate, and in their criteria for accepting a referral. Again some of them are still quite religious, and while this attitude may be a source of comfort to some people, it can have the opposite effect on others, and the pressure on the patient can be unwelcome and disturbing. So it is important when applying for hospice services to understand that you have a choice in the process, and the earlier you make contact, the more you will be able to choose, and make decisions about whether to accept what is on offer.

Dave and Jan, after her diagnosis of cancer, applied to the local hospice and went to have a look round at the facilities on offer to them. They were a gregarious couple who lived very simply, and spent most of their money on travel. They were not at all comfortable with the first place they saw, which seemed very posh to them. They were fortunate in finding, and being accepted by, an NHS specialist unit for palliative care, where they quickly felt at home, and were accepted as being within the limited area covered by the unit. With the way some services are currently funded, boundary limitations can be a problem, but it is always worth investigating all the services on offer in the area. Jan never needed care as an inpatient, but was appreciative of the care given by the social worker there, with whom she had a good rapport, and who was there for her throughout her illness, often only on the end of the phone. With their support she managed a last good holiday, which was something she had never imagined after she was told she had a short time to live.

Graham, who had the diagnosis of a rapidly progressive neurological disease at the age of thirty-three, was rejected by all the local hospice services because his need, as he saw it, was to have a bath in comfort. He was becoming increasingly immobile, but being young and fit and well built, he had a less obvious rate of muscle wasting, and so he continued to look extremely well. The local hospice, unable to appreciate the seriousness of his condition, did not accept him for their day-care services. He was fortunate enough to find a small day hospice a little further away, which understood the disease and recognised his need, and which gave him a bath and washed his hair, and provided very gentle physiotherapy each week for one day.

This also meant that he was being monitored by professionals regularly, which was a source of comfort to his wife, as well as him, and occasional changes in medication were suggested, to keep him comfortable. While the staff washed him, they also gave him the opportunity to talk, and when the talking days were over, he knew he was with people who knew him, and had a good idea of how he was feeling. It added quality to his life and to that of his family.

So perhaps the most important things to remember are that each person has a right to look for what they feel they need. No one has to accept services prescribed by other people if these are not what they want. If one option does not feel comfortable it can be put aside and considered at a later date.

Finding Other Services to Help

At this point it should be noted that there are other ways of receiving extra help at times of particular stress. Marie Curie Cancer Care is a charity that, in partnership with the local health service, provides nursing care at home for people with cancer, at times of severe stress in the last stages of the disease.

This is free to the patient. There are nurses of all grades in most areas in England, Northern Ireland, Wales and Scotland. In some areas Marie Curie nurses are used for other illnesses, while being paid for wholly by the local health services.

Local authorities also give help with home nursing, and again the district nurse and the GP will be able to access this. To find details of local services, see the help numbers at the end of this book.

Chapter Four

Making Decisions About Work

One assumption is that with a diagnosis of a disease from which one may die, the only thing to do is to give up work immediately. For some people, especially if they do not enjoy their work, and have the money, and have no family responsibilities; or if they receive an offer of early retirement or redundancy from the company, this may be the best solution. This is a decision that needs careful thought. In a good working environment, a sympathetic human resources person, or a trade union official should be consulted before any decision is made about retiring, or stopping work. There is no need to decide instantly – the wrong decision can mean the difference between leaving the family in a secure place, or worried about keeping their home and managing in the future.

There is a general belief that if someone has a life-threatening illness they will want to climb a mountain, or visit a distant country, or have a dream holiday. The truth is that most people want to live the same life they have always lived, at least initially, while they think things over. People do not always have hobbies, and it can be difficult to fill time when faced with an unplanned retirement. Whatever the decision, it is important for them to make it in their own time, without a lot of pressure.

Many people who work from home find they can continue to work at a slower pace, and perhaps in a slightly different field, and many employers are very helpful in supporting someone to stay active as long as they can.

Chris, an ambitious and single-minded bachelor aged thirty-nine, worked for a large banking organisation that, when he developed lung cancer, was prepared to assist him in his desire to remain employed. The journey to work was what exhausted him, and if he could avoid that he felt he could work for much longer. However he had to develop and promote the idea of working with a computer in his own home, and the bank was happy to give support. He was able to work in a slightly different area of banking for some time until he decided he no longer wanted to do so, and stopped of his own accord.

Helen managed to continue teaching after she developed motor neurone disease. Although her voice was affected early on, she used a small microphone and managed for two complete school terms, in order to see her students through their examinations. The class did very well overall, and the students made a major fundraising effort for a holiday for her, after she left. Many of them kept in touch with her over the summer holidays, and as her voice became much weaker she continued giving help to many of them, via the internet.

When Work is Not Possible

It is very hard for someone who has had a very physical job and then becomes ill. Greg, aged seventy, a widower for many years, was a gardener until he became ill. He had secondary cancer of the bone, which limited his activities, so he spent a large part of the summer sitting in the front garden, getting acquainted with some of the neighbours that he had hardly ever seen before, and offering tips on their gardens, which were much appreciated.

It takes courage to accept such a change in circumstances. If someone has a skill or craft that can be used no matter how disabled they may be, they will find a new pride in being able to share the knowledge they have acquired over many years.

Paula, aged sixty-three, had always loved sewing, and sewed all her married life, for friends, family, and charity. She found, after she became ill, that she could not concentrate as she once had on the intricate and detailed and beautiful garments she loved to make. However, she had a wealth of scraps left from ten years of sewing, and she started to make very simple squares of machine-stitched patchwork. These she made into cushion covers. Everyone wanted one and the requests poured in. She could work for only a short time as she became more tired, but she rarely missed working at some time in the day. She asked for a donation to her favourite charity for each one she made, and soon found she used up her store of material scraps, then people started bringing their scraps to her. Today, ten years later, her cushions hold pride of place in the homes of her friends and family, and many of the professionals who were involved in her care.

For many people there is no spare energy for hobbies, or jobs, and it is very hard to sit and accept the feelings of being useless after a busy, active and useful life. Some people find it impossible to accept a changed lifestyle, and they mourn the losses they are forced to face daily. Others can find great pleasure in very simple activities, which give satisfaction to them while in no way replacing the work or hobby they once enjoyed.

Eddie began to read again, aged seventy-four, having lost the habit over the years. With reading came a reawakened interest in astronomy. He became quite knowledgeable, and was always delighted if it was a cloudless night, and he could watch the sky from his window. It took little energy, and he was surprised at the pleasure he received from such a simple hobby.

Dick, aged seventy-nine, and an old soldier, discovered a small veterans group in the local workman's club, and met with them regularly to talk about his days in the army, and the winter passed quickly for him. As he became weaker, and less able to make the short journey, some of the little group started to come to him instead. At least once a week, most weeks, he had two or three people squashed in his tiny flat, reliving old memories.

Some people feel they have no skills that can be adapted. Joe was over eighty when his cancer finally stopped him working with the horses that had filled his life for so long. Unable to read well, and with poor eyesight, it seemed that he had no way to fill the increasing void. He sat by the fire all winter, and outside by the door for his last summer. He would have been surprised by how many people still remember him for his calm, accepting, quiet cheerfulness. He said he thought about his life, and relived the events of the last eight decades. He never grumbled or felt hard done by. Anyone speaking to him was affected by his spirit, and felt lifted by the gentle old man.

Kumar, dying rapidly from a neurological disease, found it very hard to use his skills on the computer, after his hands became severely affected. His small daughter, aged twelve, was a source of delight to him, his wife and his many visitors, as she took over the keyboard for him. In doing so she became very close to him, sharing in his care to an extent that he would never have considered possible only a short while before. She was, at the same time, building a store of memories to help her when he had died, and an expertise for her future.

Joy was a schoolteacher when she developed motor neurone disease affecting her upper limbs and voice, and cutting her career short. Her husband was reaching retirement age, her children settled and married, and she was planning another ten years in a job she loved. Unprepared for early retirement and looking forward to some promotion and advancement in her work, she was plunged into despair. Her school pupils were very sad when she told them she would have to leave and why. Interestingly the children did not seem unduly upset over the details of her disease, and in fact they were curious, as children often are, and asked very searching questions about the practicalities and the way the nerves in their bodies worked. A representative from the charity associated with the disease was asked to talk to them and was impressed with the quality of their questions. These children were all of junior-school age.

Joy was therefore delighted when a shy deputation from the school brought round three bird tables, and a bag of bird feed, with a written agreement that someone would refill the bird tables, three times a week. She accepted the offer with gratitude and amusement. Soon however she began to take an interest in wildlife, which she enjoyed for the rest of her illness. Other people added to her collection, with nesting boxes, hedgehog houses, and books on foxes. She became an enthusiast, and delighted her friends with her observations, and her increasing knowledge. When she was unable to speak she used her computer to link up with other enthusiastic nature watchers, and also to send regular letters to her former pupils about the wildlife she identified. She lived long enough to see a pond built for her by her friends and family, which was a huge source of fun, and a permanent memorial to her courage and enthusiasm afterwards.

Ben was a lonely man who did not welcome company, but sat silently watching others. Having seen the handicrafts employed at the hospice, he redeveloped the skills of tatting he learned as a child, and made some beautiful tablecloths from this form of lacework.

Janet started making up photo albums from the pile of photos that had been taken over the years. She could remember, better than most, the details of dates, times and locations. She sorted them and threw many out, and became absorbed in her hobby for hours on end. Her patience was very much appreciated by her family when they came to look through them, many months after she died.

This kind of activity can be immensely interesting for the person doing the sorting, and very rewarding for future generations. It is a task that is often left until it is too late. Family history can so easily disappear as new generations grow up. The friends and relatives in unsorted and unlabelled old photos lose significance, and are strangers to the younger members of the family.

If something can be found to interest someone who is suddenly disabled and housebound, it makes a great difference to the quality of life for everyone. Not everyone has the facilities to make a pond. And not everyone has the interest in wildlife that Joy had. But there is the potential for most people to develop a hobby of some sort, however small.

Take Your Time on Decisions and get Financial Advice

What is important is that nothing is decided in haste, and that if someone wants to continue work for as long as possible that they are given the opportunity to do so. Sadly, this may be outside their control as some companies push for early retirement, or insist on prolonged sick leave, rather than face the appearance of a sick person in the workplace. If there is real pressure then the only course is to make sure that the family and patient get the best financial agreement possible. The first questions about the possibility of continuing working should be to the specialist, because he or she will have seen this kind of situation many times before, and will have an educated opinion. Ask the questions, get a sense of the level of interest and support the specialist is showing, and then think about the answers for a while. Here again the specialist organisation, if there is one, can be a great help because of the broad experience garnered in similar situations.

If the workplace proves unhelpful in advising on this decision, then the trade union or human resources department should act in the patient's interests. If they do not then the Citizens Advice Bureau or the hospital specialist should be able to suggest a further source of help. See the Appendix in this book for more sources.

Chapter Five

How Much to Tell the Children?

In the early days following a diagnosis children in the house are often ignored, though the younger they are the more concerned everyone will be about them. This concern often shows itself by pretending that there is nothing wrong at all. Small children have very sensitive antennae in times of crisis. They quickly know that something is wrong. And they soon learn that no one is acknowledging it. They are also adept at colluding with adults to pretend that everything is all right.

It is very hard indeed for parents to give a child the feeling that it is all right to ask open questions, when the parents are in such crisis. And it may be that the child has been protected from the awareness of tragedy, until this crisis.

It is a mistake to lie to children because life-and-death lies will always be discovered in the end. Even very small children know when they are being deceived, and will either be very quiet and resigned, or will play up and generally be naughty and unmanageable. If they are given truthful answers to their questions they may still have difficult times, but they are less likely to have long-term problems after the experience.

It is also a mistake to spoil the children in an attempt

to keep them happy. Children need boundaries. They do not like a lot of change. If they are allowed to run riot they feel 'out of control' and unsupported. It is wiser to keep to the general house rules, whatever they were before the parent was ill. Bedtimes, watching television, mealtimes, all contribute to a feeling of normality.

Special Care for Very Small Children

With very tiny children it is not possible to make very detailed explanations, but they can usually understand that Mummy or Daddy is ill. They are rarely as aware of the physical change in people, and they are not as frightened by physical deterioration, as are many adults. Nor are they as frightened by clinical activities like intravenous infusions (tubes in the arm or neck), or radiation burns, or operation scars. They are usually just interested. However, they will often overhear comments by adults, and this is what can be frightening for them. So it is important to make time to answer honestly (within reason) any questions they may ask. They may need to ask the same question repeatedly, and of more than one person, until they have accepted the answer. They often need a lot of reassurance that it is not their fault that Mummy, or whoever, is ill. When something bad happens to a close family member, a child will often immediately conclude that they have been the cause of the problem. Small children often say they wish they had another mother, or say 'I hate you' to a little sibling, and then assume responsibility for anything bad that might happen afterwards. Like adults they look for a reason, and like adults, they feel to blame.

It is also especially important to emphasise that there will always be someone there to look after them, since small children are very aware that they are helpless, and need grownups to care for them. After the initial interest, they usually accept the situation very calmly, often because they cannot understand the finality of death until they are much older, perhaps as old as ten or eleven.

A visiting district nurse was asked by Ruth, aged five years, 'My mummy is very ill, did you know that?'

She was told, 'Yes, that is why I am here, to help look after her.'

Ruth then said, 'Are you going to make her better?'

She was told sadly that the nurse could not do that.

Ruth's next question was, 'Whose fault is it? Was it something I did?'

The nurse was able to reassure her very definitely that it was not her fault, and that she could not make anyone ill: no one could do that, and no one could possibly be to blame. The nurse emphasised that no one was cross with Ruth, but that everyone was sad and worried about her mummy, and that was why they seemed cross sometimes. The little girl needed to be reminded of this regularly throughout her mother's illness, but she accepted the gradual loss of weight, and the deterioration of her mother as time went by, without panic, and without anxiety, but with an understanding that seemed very mature. Her only comment on the loss of weight was that Mummy was getting smaller and smaller, like the children in some of the news on television. She was told that her mummy just could not eat, even food she really liked, unlike the children on the news on television, who could eat but had no food. And yes, her mummy was getting smaller and smaller. Ruth did not appear to be worried about this.

As time went by, she seemed to accept that her mother would die, but she still asked, 'Will Mummy come back for Christmas?' and people found it hard to keep telling her that Mummy would never be able to come back, however much she wanted to. Small children simply cannot understand the concept of dying being forever.

The Continuing Effects of Our Own Childhood

Alan was ten when his father died. He had awful memories of the illness and the day his father was taken sobbing in pain to the hospital, never to be seen again. He was assured in the early stages of his father's illness that it was not serious, and in those days this was the common practice. No one told him when the illness became serious, and he never asked, because he had no one to ask. He was given extra treats, sweets and toys and generally anything that would keep him occupied and quiet. He had a very strong belief for many years that he had made his father ill, because he was a very lively and mischievous little boy, who was often in trouble. He grew up with a great fear of death, and especially death from cancer. He slept with a light on, until he married at twenty-three. When he was diagnosed with lung cancer at forty-one, and told he would not live much longer than eighteen months, he was absolutely determined, despite the total shock of such a diagnosis, not to repeat the same mistakes with his own children. His wife was a calm and supportive woman, but they both had to contend with his mother, who was now reliving her previous experience, but this time with her only son. She was grief-stricken, but she was also very sure that she was the expert in this situation.

At the very beginning Alan and Betty told their daughters, of eight and ten, that he had a very serious illness. To his surprise, they immediately asked if it was AIDS, and he realised that they had been having some questions already, and were aware of something badly wrong. He told them it was cancer. They asked many questions, which he told them honestly he could not answer at that time. He said he wanted very much to live a long time, and he would do his best with the help of the hospital, but no one knew what might happen. He said it was nobody's fault that these things happen. He did wish he had never smoked, but no one made him smoke, and he had just liked doing it. After the initial discussion the girls asked very few questions, just how he was feeling every now and then. They felt able to be open at school with friends who also knew him. Several times they told Betty that they didn't want him to die, and she agreed and cried with them, but said they must carry on hoping. The discussions were in the main open and free between the family, though his mother could never bring herself to mention the word.

Trying to Meet the Needs of the Whole Family

With older children it is a question of taking things at whatever pace seems right for them. Kate, a single mum for more than ten years, lived with her three children. Ann, the eldest at nineteen, was out at work and often seemed unaware of the problems at home. Jane, aged seventeen, was in the middle of her exams, and very preoccupied. Clare, at twelve, became the main carer, since she was home for the greatest period each day, and she worried and fretted, and was superficially the most frightened. In the aftermath of the diagnosis, it took a lot of effort on the part of the mother, her sister and the district nurse to talk to the girls individually. Without putting blame or pressure on any of the children, they tried to get each one to share their understanding of the situation, and then to see how they could offer some support. Fortunately, Kate realised quite early on that each of her children was coping with her fears in her own way, though by apparently denying her illness they all appeared to be very selfish. It is not at all uncommon for teenagers to act like this. Blaming and accusing them does not make them more thoughtful, because they are usually very frightened, and only want to run away.

If the situation is discussed at an early stage, and no one is excluded or over-protected, then there is time to build relationships and make changes that may become impossible at a later date. Kate felt that anything was better than angry confrontations, and accusations of selfishness, especially when she felt so weak and ill.

Sometimes in this kind of situation a good friend can be helpful with the children, but if not, it is worth talking to the school, or perhaps a counsellor, or tutor at college. At the start of a serious illness, it is well worth informing the school or college about the situation, so that someone is aware of any stress the student is experiencing. Spouses and partners are not often able to be objective enough to see through the children's mixed emotions, while simultaneously coping with their own grief. There is a lot of support from some of the charities. There are some addresses in the Appendix of this book.

The trouble can become worse when the child who is seen to be having the behavioural problem becomes the focus of all the attention. The child then inevitably feels that all the pressure is on him or her, and is aware of being talked about and grumbled about freely, within the family circle. Even an outsider can sometimes see that one child within the family is reacting in such an extreme way, that the focus of the family is on that one child, and it is being blamed for all the problems. The situation can then become a sort of ganging-up, and the child feels absolutely isolated. It is important to recognise that all children have their own fears, and the only way to express that fear is through disruptive behaviour. It helps if they have someone of their own to talk to, who will respect their privacy and their confidence, and understand them.

Outside Help Can be Useful

Some older children become parental, trying in any way possible to have some control over this uncontrollable part of their lives. The best way to handle difficult behaviour is to talk about it, and if this is not possible within the family, the solution is to ask for outside help.

A close relationship with a teacher was a great support to Mark, at fifteen, when his mother was dying. She had received her diagnosis after a long and depressing period of investigations, and was therefore fairly ill by the time she contacted the school. A rather distant older father meant that Mark had been used to keeping all his fears to himself since he was a small boy. A direct question from his sports teacher seemed to him at first quite invasive and brutal. 'I understand your mother is very ill, Mark? How are things for you at home?' He responded very curtly. However when the teacher told him the same thing had happened to him at the same age, Mark felt able to talk to him, and the teacher was able to listen without offering advice. He also understood Mark's need to play an aggressive game of tennis, or squash, when life seemed particularly difficult. He proved a huge support until, and after, Mark's mother died. His father never discussed her illness with him, so he valued the support from his teacher.

Sometimes local organisations offer support, sometimes charities, and sometimes it has to be paid for, when a private counsellor is contacted. A charity concerned with the disease or illness may be able to fund the help, if it is impossible within the family. And often, with the onset of unexpected illness when someone is young, the family may not have the financial resources in hand to cope with all the demands they will meet. It is hard to learn to ask for help, and hard to accept the help, but it is even harder to watch carefully conserved finances vanishing fast.

Consider Other Therapy

When the sick parent is hardly more than a child itself, the problems can seem overwhelming. Lucy was given a neurological diagnosis, which, at only twenty-one years of age, was very rapid and very debilitating. She was immature for her age, in spite of an early marriage and a young family of two toddlers. She was severely handicapped early on by the disease, but received a diagnosis only after a long delay. A close friend was aware of her need to do something creative, and asked for some funding from a local support group, for Lucy to have some sessions of art therapy. At first, it seemed an impossible proposition, since she had never shown any aptitude for art. However she eventually had twelve sessions with an art therapist, and produced some good work with her, which helped her greatly in those early days to come to terms with all that was happening to her. This was a wonderful therapy for her, and she could leave behind a tangible and thoughtful gift. At the very least her children would one day be able to learn something of the mother they had no time to get to know.

Art as a way of expressing emotions is fairly new in current thinking, and there are few therapists around who have been trained in this skill. However just using pen or paint is a relaxing hobby for many people, and many day centres and hospices have regular art sessions for their patients. Small children who are ill themselves, or have parents or siblings who are ill, can often draw feelings better than they can describe them. Elisabeth Kübler-Ross has written about art for terminally ill children with great effect, as well as books about death and loss for children and adults.

Children Who Have Parents With Long-term Illness

Children can find long-term illness very hard to deal with. Phil, aged six, had no memory of his mother Anne ever being well. She had cancer for most of his young life. His strongest relationship was with his twelve-year-old sister

Lyn, who became his main carer, doing school runs between her lessons, and taking Phil everywhere with her. When Phil finally realised that Anne was going to leave them forever, he pleaded with his dad to get them a proper mother quickly, so he could bring friends home to play like the other children. His comments caused great pain to the family, and it was hard for them to respond to him calmly. But, as a small child he simply wanted to be like everyone else. It was Anne who most understood his needs, and was able to agree with him that his next mother should be a well one.

There cannot be one answer for all the different attitudes children can display, but as long as children or young people are respected and given truthful answers they will be able to make their own sense of what is happening. Mistakes will be made, but an honest approach means that when a mistake has been made, it is easy to say 'I really should have done/said this' or 'I'm sorry I didn't do this or understand that or realise why this happened.' The child will know he or she can ask any questions, and everyone is ready to help and support. Sometimes a book can open up the subject for a child, and some are listed at the end of this one.

There is one aspect of looking after children in the case of parental illness that is easily overlooked, but that is critical when a parent is unable to give the child full attention. This is the time when a vulnerable child can easily be 'comforted' and 'befriended' by the kind of person who is on the lookout for vulnerable children. In the past this has not been a subject that was openly discussed, or even frequently reported by the victims, and so there has not been much knowledge about the level of this crime. However, today there is a great deal of information about paedophiles in the popular press, and we are beginning to realise how very often it has occurred in the past. This makes it easy to become suspicious of all strangers who show an interest in a child. The sad fact is that most children are approached by a family member, whom they know and trust, and usually one who seems the least likely to harm them.

Paedophiles look just like any other person. They can be any age, and of either sex. If they looked dangerous and frightening, the children would run away from them, and parents would keep their children away from them. Often these people appear kind and friendly and full of fun, which is just what a child who is worried or confused, or apprehensive, will respond to most easily. Children who are used to a lot of attention from a parent may be missing that focussed love and attention and pride and interest in their achievements. They could respond to someone who seems to offer the same warmth.

However, these are evil and manipulative people who will use any situation to gain access to a child, and it is easy, in the stress of the moment, for a parent to accept gratefully the help, especially if they know the person offering it.

So parents and family should be aware of this particular danger. However honest the parent may feel their relationship is with the children, no one can be sure that their child will feel safe enough to tell them about something so frightening. Many children are taught to be polite to adults, and as a result they find it hard to reject adults who behave strangely, however inappropriately, because they feel they are being rude. Sometimes the child may feel guilty, or have been threatened, or feel he or she may not be believed. Or may be so shocked as to be unable to find the words to describe what has happened. If something happens to you that is new and strange, you find it hard to believe it yourself. It is even harder to describe it to someone else, and if the abuser tells you this is the way everyone behaves, it is even harder to question anyone else.

A relative or close friend who suddenly becomes very close to a child, and spends a lot of time with the child, is not necessarily a danger, and is more likely to be a great support to the child, and help out massively with the family dynamics. However, parents and workers within the family should be aware of the chance, however remote, of a child turning to an adult who will do harm.

A child wanting to lock the bedroom door, wanting to sleep with a sibling, seeming distant, changing in responses to someone, can all be small signs that something is amiss. Asking questions, 'Why are you scared of someone coming into your room?' or 'Do you like so-and-so?' or 'What did you do with so-and-so this afternoon?' Ask questions and listen carefully to the reply. And try not to appear too anxious or suspicious, so that the child is not made worried by your attitude, or is made frightened to meet new people.

The only thing anyone can do is to be aware of the possibility, encourage the child to talk whenever possible, and listen and observe any changes in behaviour, however small. Paedophiles usually take time to groom their victims, and this is when it may be possible to see any small changes in the behaviour of the child.

Helpful Books for Children to Read

This list is reproduced at the end of the book:

Beginnings and Endings With Lifetimes in Between, by Bryan Mellonie and Robert Ingpen, ISBN 1-85028-038X. A Dragon's World Ltd Imprint.
When Uncle Bob Died, by Althea, published by Dinosaur Publications, ISBN 0-85122-727-9.
Gran's Grave, by Wendy Green, published by Lion Press, ISBN 0-7459-1556-6.
The Tenth Good Thing about Barney, by Judith Viorst, published by Aladdin Paperbacks, ISBN 0-689-71203-0.

Am I still a Sister? by Alicia M Sims, published by Gilgal Publications, ISBN 0-9618995-0-6.

Badger's Parting Gifts, by S Varley, published by Picture Lion.

The Fall of Freddie the Leaf, by Leo Buscaglia, published by Slack, ISBN 0-8050-1064-5.

Waterbugs and Dragonflies, by D Stickney, published by London Mowbray.

How it Feels When a Parent Dies, by Jill Krementz, published by Gollancz, ISBN 0-575-05183-3.

Goodbye Mog, by Judith Kerr, published by Collins Children's Books.

Name all the Animals, by Alison Smith, published by Shuber.

Chapter Six

Caring for the Carer

For many people the physical work involved in caring for someone at home, however hard, is nothing compared with the anguish of never being able to make things better, to provide all the answers. Washing, cooking and cleaning are almost the easy part. Watching a beloved person gradually changing, losing hope, feeling weaker, coping with so much change, is the hardest part of the whole situation. And no one else can understand, unless they too have been in the same place. That is why so much benefit can be derived from having the right emotional as well as physical support at the right time.

Some carers manage to remain calm, and conceal their feelings with apparent ease. For some, this is difficult, if not impossible.

Again, very few people will appreciate the overall effort involved in caring for someone at home. In a home that has been looked after by two people, illness almost always involves learning new skills, and managing new household chores. Even for the few who can afford full-time live-in care, and are surrounded with love and support, it is still exhausting.

All of the suggestions in this book about hygiene and

appearance and adequate fluid intake apply equally to carers, who have to remain healthy, because they are the lynchpin of the whole situation. This chapter looks particularly at the carer.

It is also important to remember that self-image can vary day to day, and if you are stressed and exhausted it is easy to forget to care for yourself, and to become unkempt and neglected, never eating proper meals or having a good rest. Apart from anything else, this is hard for the patient to observe since inevitably they will feel very responsible.

As we have seen, one thing that people outside the home often do not realise, especially the professionals, is how hard the carer finds it to keep pace with all there is to do. Many carers worry because they feel they are constantly living in a mess. They feel ashamed of the house, which they think never gets properly cleaned. Caring for someone all day is time-consuming and exhausting. Someone who has been organised and efficient all their life cannot believe they can get so behind with their chores. When you are a carer, you have to be ready to adapt continually to other people's needs. You feel that your life is never your own anymore. This often adds to the feeling of inadequacy when, after some time looking after someone, there is still no organisation, and the house is still a mess. And if the carer is a man, who has never been involved with the housekeeping, he will find it hard to cope with the many varied aspects of a job of which he has no experience.

The carer can also lose their former role within the family and the community. Few people imagine becoming a full-time carer. They may have plans of their own for the future, perhaps when the children are grown, or the mortgage paid. They rarely anticipate being so helpless in the face of huge life changes. It is not unusual to want desperately to run away. The person who is ill has no choice about running away, but for the carer the choices may seem quite impossible. They can see their life fading into oblivion until they are too old to pick up the pieces.

They need constant reassurance that they are doing a good job. It is easy for visitors to notice and even comment to each other that the house is a mess, and the ironing not done. That is why any offer of help is appreciated, even if it takes a while to persuade someone to accept the help. Anyone who has spent a few hours a day visiting a friend in hospital soon realises how tired they can get. Looking after someone at home is much harder.

What Friends Can Do to Help

- Do give encouragement and praise. These are often not given and cost very little effort. But do mean what is said. Imagine yourself coping with the same situation. Insincerity is not a support.

- Do ask how someone feels, and really want to hear the answer. The carer needs to talk sometimes, and be listened to.

- Depending on how the suggestion is taken, do offer to wash up a cup after a drink. Little things like changing the water, wiping a surface, spending time with the patient, so that the carer can get upstairs to tidy up or pop to the shop or just sit and read the paper, can make a huge difference.

- Do NOT repeat conversations with either the carer or the patient to people outside. If they want something repeated they will do it themselves. It is incredibly hurtful to find that one is the subject of gossip, however kindly it is meant. It is all too easy to become the 'voice of the visitor'. Gossip has a nasty way of growing. Even if it is meant kindly, no one likes to be the topic of conversation and scrutiny.

This is especially important if the carer has had a grumble about the professional team, or the sick person. After giving way to a grumble, the carer will usually feel guilty enough, without wondering whether they are being judged and criticised.

There is no need to take gifts along daily, but here are some ideas for useful presents. The carer often appreciates a gift that can be shared, and is not meant only for the patient.

Some of these ideas are small and cheap and some are larger and more suitable for two or three people to give on a special occasion—

- Non-allergic soaps, or non-perfumed refreshing wipes. If it is known that someone has a favourite perfume, then that is a nice gift, otherwise it is better to choose a neutral non-perfumed gift, especially when someone has a problem with breathing.
- Shampoos are often useful gifts.
- Hand creams of all sorts are appreciated, as both the carer and the patient can develop very dry skin. (Again do not give strongly perfumed creams unless you are very sure of your choice.)
- Talcum powder has the disadvantage of clogging in creases and can make the skin sore, unless you know someone has always used it, and still does.
- Fruit juices or herbal teas in small sachets, so that small quantities can be tried out. Or savoury drinks like Bovril or beef tea.
- A home visit from a hairdresser or a chiropodist. Or a massage from an aromatherapist – perhaps a hand massage, or foot massage, if someone is very weak, or has not had one before.
- Homemade soup, or a special meal in cool weather, or some fresh fruit juice or fruit salad in hot weather.

It is often hard for a carer to find time to make a special effort with meals, and something that is tasty and nutritious (and prepared by another person) is a real luxury.

- Books or magazines that are easy to hold, and that refer to a particular interest like cars or gardening.
- Small cards for 'Thank you' notes that save the carer time as well.
- Miniature bottles of wine or sherry are often appreciated and can act as an aperitif for indifferent appetites, and can be enjoyed by both patient and carer.
- Flowers or pot plants are often appreciated as an illness progresses, since after the initial shock of diagnosis people often stop bringing them. It is always worth checking on space available, and the quantity of flowers already in the house.
- Luxury rubber gloves for the carer. The carer also often appreciates the chance of a hand or foot massage as well, and often a double booking can be done at a special rate.
- Tapes or CDs if someone has a specific interest in music or cannot read easily due to fatigue or poor eyesight. They can be bought or loaned.
- Small fans in hot weather, or heaters in cold weather, can be cheaply bought or even loaned. Suggestions like these are useful ahead of time, anticipating a change in temperature, as carers often find it hard thinking ahead when there is so much to do.
- Lightweight fleeces and blankets that are portable and easy to use in many different circumstances as well as being easy to wash and dry.
- Microwaveable hot water bottles or fragrant pads if it is cold, or to ease an aching back.

- Small towels are always useful, as large towels are heavy and unwieldy, especially for use in bed. Hair-washing turbans are often appreciated, as are extra tea towels. Also having someone bed-bound for a while causes quite a lot of extra washing and washing-up.

- Sometimes a couple will appreciate some new mugs or cups, as having a stream of visitors, and perhaps professional carers coming and going, puts a strain on limited crockery supplies.

- A box of nice biscuits also means the carer can offer them round, without having to think about providing them.

- As we have already said it is possible to give generously without spending a lot of money. Doing something like cutting a lawn, weeding a flowerbed, collecting some washing, doing some ironing, washing up, are all gifts that make a difference. There is no need to take home all the washing – just taking some of the burden off the shoulders of the main carer makes a huge contribution to their feeling of emotional and physical support. It is really a question of keeping aware of what is waiting to be done, and doing it without taking over and intruding.

- Many sick people do not want chocolates or rich foods, but a small box to tuck away for special moments is often a great treat. It is a gift that has to be thought out because, for example, giving chocolate to a chocoholic carer, who cannot keep them for more than an hour, may not be appreciated. In that case, perhaps just taking a tiny box with two or three in it is a thoughtful gesture.

- Some people are embarrassed about physical contact, and would hate to have a friend offer to cream their feet. But if the offer is made, and there is time to consider it, and the giver is quite comfortable with the action, it is a wonderful experience and very relaxing, especially as skin on legs and feet becomes very dry and itchy after a while in bed.

- Herbal deodorants are also a personal gift, but if given in the right way they are much appreciated, as they usually cause no irritation, and are not sticky. And often the carer has no time to shop around and research products on the market.

- An offer of shopping help is usually appreciated. The offer of a lift to the supermarket on a quiet day is a great help, depending on the carer. Sometimes the greatest help is to offer to stay with the person who is ill, so that the carer can shop at their leisure for once. Making the offer flexible so that it can be adapted to the needs of the carer is always appreciated.

- Sometimes a gesture like taking out the dustbin for the collection, and bringing it in after collection, seems very small and inadequate, and yet makes a tremendous difference to the carer. Watching garden rubbish or old newspapers build up can be a source of anxiety out of all proportion to someone already anxious and stressed.

- NEVER VISIT IF YOU HAVE A COLD OR A SORE THROAT. It is very worrying for a carer to sit and watch someone coughing over them or their patient. In fact, people who are so ill do not often seem to catch colds and coughs, but they do feel very vulnerable. And the carer, stressed and tired, may be very vulnerable to infection, so make a phone call instead.

Most of all make it plain that any offer of help is made because you have a genuine desire to do so, and a genuine awareness of, and admiration for, the difficulties involved in caring for someone at home. And also because you care for them, and want to show it by being part of all that is happening to them at such a time.

Lastly, be aware that many children become carers, almost without anyone noticing. There are support services for children (see Appendix), but everyone can be supportive by being aware that the child will want to help, and not allowing him or her to work so hard that they have no other life. It is too easy to forget that children especially may not complain at all, and therefore shoulder more and more of the burden of care. It may be hard to persuade them to take time out to be a child, and it may take a visitor to the house to identify the situation, and step in to help.

Chapter Seven

Looking at Ways in Which Everyone Can Help

It is helpful for the person at the centre of the situation, the patient, to feel that he or she is contributing something other than grief to the family. Sometimes, this means asking friends to step in. This can be hard at first, though usually friends and family are only too grateful to be able to help. The nature of the help depends upon the local area, and the access to facilities, as well as the courage to ask.

Eric and Carol were very close, and had a wide circle of friends to call upon. Initially, they found it hard to ask for what they saw as favours. With professional help, and the persistence of family and friends, they were able to realise that when help was offered it was foolish to reject any opportunity to make life easier. They were finally able to come to an arrangement whereby Eric invited a friend round weekly to watch football on the TV (sometimes recorded for him) and Carol had a specific four hours or so to go to the theatre, or indulge in what she called 'retail therapy'. Instead of using that time to catch up on vital business, she managed to save it for pleasure. Friends enjoyed the time with Eric and were glad to feel they were able to do something constructive at the same time.

If the idea of time out is accepted from the very beginning, then it is not too hard to adapt the length and quality of the time available. It is a much harder idea if, from the beginning, the carer has been on call without a break, because they then feel as if they are failing in their duty of care. Equally the patient may also feel responsible for causing the exhaustion, and the intolerable situation, and then both parties are left feeling guilty.

As people become more ill, they may become more demanding, and less appreciative of another point of view. Being confined to one room limits perspective. It is easy to resent the health that other people take for granted. Even as short a time as three weeks in one room makes a difference. There is less to talk about, because the patient is not doing anything interesting, and the carer cannot either. Some women can knit or sew for short periods, but many men simply fret, though Ben (mentioned in Chapter Four), a former sailor and a 'tough macho man', came into his own when he was forced to take to his bed. His mother had taught him 'tatting' when he was a very small boy, though he had not thought about it for fifty years. When he saw a woman sewing in the day-care hospice he asked to join in, and quickly regained his skill and interest. Thereafter his hobby filled his days. He discovered that he was a natural extrovert, instead of the loner he had appeared to be, and he enjoyed the teasing that came his way, as well as completing some beautiful lace cloths.

People find it harder to accept new people who did not know them before they were ill. They may feel they have lost their whole personality: their status if they had a job, their role within the family, their standing among friends. A stranger cannot imagine the young personality and will only be able to relate to the present one. Old friends can see beyond the image of the sick person.

The longer one is ill, the harder it becomes to act

unselfishly, even to the point of accepting the need for giving a carer a break. And of course exhaustion limits the patience required for both the carer and the patient, in training someone new into the usual routine.

The carer may resent what seems to be the apparent selfishness of the patient, and yet may even feel guilty about the resentment.

In other words, the idea of pacing out the time and stress makes the whole situation much easier. If someone tries to be all things to all people, the stress is immense, and no single human being can do this for a long period. Having that understanding from the very beginning goes a long way towards preventing exhaustion and depression, and the feeling that one cannot go on any longer. It also gives balance to the relationship, in that both carer and patient are considering each other, as well as themselves. And a change of activity gives an opportunity for sharing new experiences.

Responding to the Attitudes of Other People

It cannot be said too often that looking after someone at home is much more than a full-time job. Friends, family and professional carers see only a fraction of the effort that is required by the main carer. A nurse who stays with the patient for a full twelve-hour shift has a better idea of the weariness that can be experienced, but even they can then go home to sleep and to have time off. A carer who lives with the sick person has to become used to broken nights as well as long and busy days. It is easy to feel as if you are on a treadmill.

Many carers are frustrated by the lack of understanding by those closest to them. There is no point at all in hoping that anyone will understand, because they cannot. Most people stay for a few hours and see a small part of the whole picture. The professionals do their job, hope to have time for a quick chat, and they are away. Family and friends are mainly concerned with asking after the person who is ill. It is rare that the first question is 'And how are you?'

Someone who has to make a daily visit to the hospital for several weeks can appreciate how exhausting it can be to make the daily trip, keep up with the laundry and the chores at home. Most people are surprised when they first realise how very tiring this can be.

In the same way, to understand anything of the experience and the frustration of the carer at home, one has to have experienced the same situation, or observed it from close quarters.

This is another reason why it is helpful for the family to participate in the general care, because as well as relieving the main carer, the whole family appreciates the stresses, and are able to support and encourage each other. They can often see when the main carer is in need of a break, they can identify with the escalating emotions, and they can offer the kind of support that is truly helpful. It is hard to accept help when someone has been more used to giving the help than receiving it. Offering support or help often sounds like a casual or throwaway remark.

'DO GIVE ME A CALL IF THERE IS ANYTHING I CAN DO AT ANY TIME'

If the offer is meant why not make it clearly defined? For example:

'May I take this washing home with me now and I will return it later.'

'If it is fine tomorrow I will come and cut the grass.'

'I have made this meal for you both. All you need to do is pop it in the microwave.'

'I am doing a big shop on Thursday so please make a list for me to collect for you. Or can I take you with me.'

'I will visit on Wednesday and perhaps you would like to have an hour or two free to sleep or whatever and I'll stay with her/him.'

'Would the children like to come and sleep over at the weekend? We will have a barbecue on Saturday.'

★

Someone like Jeanette (Chapter Sixteen) was able to see the family draw together and support each other. She could relax and accept all the care they offered, without worrying that one was getting more tired than the others. The family worked as a team.

It is easy to advise the carer to ignore what is said by the uninformed. It is hard to forget thoughtless remarks, however casually they are spoken, if they show a lack of empathy and understanding by people from whom one would expect care and support.

Here are some examples of what not to say:

'YOU WILL COPE, YOU ARE SO STRONG'

Sometimes strength is not a choice because there is either an unacceptable alternative, or there is no alternative at all. It is an added pressure when there is an assumption that one will cope. Most carers do cope amazingly well but most also feel inadequate and fear they are not going to be able to manage. They need to be able to voice these fears.

'PUTTING A LIFT IN THE HOUSE IS NO PROBLEM AS THEY SIMPLY TAKE OUT THE CORNER OF THE CEILING IN THE SITTING ROOM AND IT MAKES VERY LITTLE MESS'

Most people have planned and decorated their house without thinking of adding a lift at some time. The thought comes as a huge shock, and is often resisted fiercely. It is not seen as a small change, but as a massive alteration, as well as an acceptance of the unthinkable. Making it sound like a minor change is to deny the significance of such an adaptation.

'THEY MAKE GOOD WHEELCHAIRS NOWADAYS'

Nobody relishes the idea of using a wheelchair, no matter how smart and modern it is. This is no comfort, neither is the mention of a good guide dog when threatened with loss of vision, nor a hearing aid if hearing loss is threatened. In any life all these changes are traumatic, even if they offer relief. Minimising them does not help. The person using the appliance may be able to make such comments in an attempt to comfort themselves, but not anyone else.

Sometimes there is no comfort that can be offered in a situation. And then it is better to say nothing at all. Silence is very helpful at times. For the person at the centre of the situation, the patient, it can help to repeat the problem several times over; they are not asking for a solution because there is none. They are simply becoming accustomed to the idea, or they are voicing their deepest fears.

'YOU HAVE A VERY GOOD FAMILY, THEY WILL BE BOUND TO HELP'

However good the family may appear, there is no assurance that they will be able to give the amount of help that is needed. Assumptions of support systems are impossible, even when the family is well known to the speaker. It is better to allow the carer to identify their sources of support.

Many families are committed to jobs, routines that are difficult if not impossible to alter. It is pointless to raise the hopes of the main carer; and it can make them feel very defensive of their family if they have to try and explain why it seems that the family are not as responsive as they might be. And many competent and resourceful people cannot cope with some aspects of illness. Making assumptions means they will appear to fail and this can cause extra grief in the family. It is kinder and much more productive to encourage and appreciate the help available.

'WE CAN HOPE FOR A MIRACLE'

Everyone hopes for a miracle. However, there are not so many on record. And few people expect one. It is very important not to lose heart but no one benefits from false optimism. If the remark comes from the patient then it does not help to dash their hopes either, but better to say something like. 'And we are all hoping for one with you,' and leave it at that.

'I READ THIS BOOK ABOUT THIS MAN WHO DID/SAW/TOOK... AND IS NOW CURED'

Again, raising false hopes does not help. Many books are very helpful indeed, and offering them as another informative source is a kind gesture. But it is not helpful to become evangelical about cures. Likewise the internet can be very informative but the information on a website is very varied and often very inaccurate, and cannot be taken as the absolute truth.

Very few people want to change their doctors unless they have been badly hurt and disillusioned by their treatment. They need to have faith in the people at the top. Undermining that confidence is not helpful, unless the family feels there has been an obvious and catastrophic neglect or mismanagement, in which case it can be very helpful to support them in assessing the right course to follow.

'YOU MUST TRY AND LOOK ON THE BRIGHT SIDE/STAY POSITIVE'

This is particularly unhelpful when someone is trying to be realistic. Of course it is easier and less distressing for visitors if they never see any signs of distress, but the carer cannot be anything but stressed by having to appear cheery and hopeful all the time. Allowing someone to be sad if they wish is very helpful.

'I KNOW JUST HOW YOU FEEL'

No one can say this even if they have been in the same situation. Each experience is different, though the feelings are often the same. It can be very irritating when people assume that they can understand absolutely. It also acts as an effective gag since there is no point in elaborating on an experience if someone is so well informed.

'YOU MUST FIGHT IT. DON'T LET THE CANCER/DISEASE, ETC. WIN'

It is not possible to 'fight' a disease. It is possible to put energy into co-operating fully with all instructions. It is possible to look at all the complementary therapies that may strengthen and support the course of the illness. It is possible to remain optimistic and hope that the treatment is going to give time and quality of life.

Telling someone to fight is a vague and at the same time a fixed position. How can anyone fight? And with what are they meant to fight? And if they do not get better does that mean they have lost? Or not tried hard enough?

None of these remarks helps. If there is nothing to say, then the best response is silence.

This does not mean that visitors should be gloomy. Silent understanding is not gloomy, and often the carer will be ready to share laughter if they feel they have been listened to, and understood.

Paul was glad to share his story about 'open wide, Daddy' with his friends when they visited (Chapter Fourteen), and Penny's furious gardening became a source of amusement to many friends, and she also enjoyed the joke (Chapter Fourteen).

Most people like to laugh, especially if they know the participants in the joke. It is also very therapeutic to have a good laugh, especially in times of extreme stress. Gloomy visitors are no help at all.

This makes it all sound very complicated to visit someone who is ill or dying. In fact most people love to see someone for short spells, and if you can be yourself, and simply try to put yourself in the position of the person you are visiting, it does not have to be too complex or difficult.

Chapter Eight

The Physical Needs of the Person Who is Ill

'Physical needs' means more than just basic bodily functions. If someone is physically uncomfortable for any reason, they will find it almost impossible to concentrate on anything else. If they do not feel clean and fresh they will find all their other symptoms unbearable. The most frequently voiced complaint following hospital admission is that people have not had a proper bath or wash.

Being unable to perform simple everyday toilet care always causes great distress and humiliation for the person who is ill. If you have never done it before, trying to wash and dress someone, however close a relationship you have with them, is time-consuming and complex. However, it can also be a time of growing intimacy, and great personal satisfaction and pleasure, if the chore can be viewed in a different way.

The first rule in caring for someone at home is to accept any professional help that is offered, even if it seems very paltry and inadequate. Once you allow a professional carer into your lives, it follows that someone outside the family is aware of a need, and is monitoring the situation. The professional carer will observe the situation, and hopefully suggest an increase in the care offered, if it is necessary, and if it is possible. And for the carer, even a short break is better than nothing.

How to Give Good Physical Care

STARTING WITH A GOOD WASH

Washing someone is quite a skilled task if they are to feel fresh, and clean, and comfortable when the carer has finished. People also vary considerably in their personal toilet needs, depending on lifestyle, facilities and habit. Some people bathe daily, some prefer a shower. Whatever the preference, it is very unlikely that help offered by Social Services will provide the level of care that the person has been used to. So the bulk of the care will usually fall upon the carer.

In the early days of a diagnosis, an extra chair in the bathroom can enable someone to manage fairly well, though it is always nice to have a helping hand to steady and reassure, if someone is weak and a little unsteady.

The main secret of a *good* wash is to have a warm room, and use hot water and plenty of it, changing it if necessary several times. Think about washing your own face, and what a good wash feels like to you. Start at the face, using firm movements, and washing behind the ears and around the neck carefully, and thoroughly. It is also important to use clean and dry towels, and again to wipe firmly, which is not the same as roughly. Men and women usually wash in very different ways. Women do not often scrub themselves as enthusiastically as men like to, and when washing other people they are inclined to pat and wash tenderly. Men however may still scrub away as if their victim has never been washed before. Jill, after having her hair washed by her partner, felt exhausted and as battered as if she had been in a car wash. This was a joke for her as she was only temporarily disabled, but it is not so funny for someone who is ill and weak.

Sometimes a person who has been used to a daily bath can manage comfortably with a 'top and tail' wash on alternate days, when they are at home and inactive for much of the time (and especially if they have to wash in bed). This means washing the face, hands, underarms and genital area and perhaps the feet. It sounds a lengthy process but is something that can be done fairly quickly if two carers are involved, and it can be fun. It is also less time-consuming, and less tiring. Soaking feet is a wonderful aid to relaxing, which can be done at any time during the day, and can be an end-of-the-day treat for both carer and patient.

A shower is probably the quickest way to have a good wash, if it is available safely, for example if there are grab rails for someone who is unsteady, and a non-slip mat, or even a stool in the shower cubicle.

A bed bath takes a certain skill, and is sadly rarely in evidence in hospitals these days. Again the room needs to be warm and the towels dry.

The patient is undressed, and covered with a warm towel, or a blanket. Starting at the top of the body, soap is applied in small areas, and then removed with a warm, soap-free flannel, and the skin dried immediately. Again use a separate washcloth for genital areas, and put the cloths in the general wash regularly, so they remain fresh. Whether the room is warm or cold, it is important never to leave someone uncovered for long periods. Pay special attention to ears and neck and underarms and creases, and dry them well.

Again a foot soak is very comforting, and can be done at the very end of the wash, while the patient has a rest and perhaps has their hair tidied.

As we said, imagine you are washing yourself, and act accordingly. Always keep the patient as dry and covered as possible as you work your way down, so that they do not become cold. It is surprising how quickly you will become very adept and competent. Giving a bed bath is a skilled and much appreciated art and can be enjoyed together, especially if the carer does not mind taking some direction at critical points. Usually the patient is able to wash his or her own private areas themselves. Chris from Chapter Four always asked his carer, 'Do you want to do my party pieces or shall I keep that pleasure for myself?' And he received some fairly smart replies from his amused carers.

Everyone has a different standard or idea about personal hygiene. What matters is that agreements are reached, and compromises made, so that the person in the centre does not feel neglected and dirty, and the carers are not stressed and exhausted. It is often hard to agree on the amount of washing someone requires. Some elderly people have not been able to manage a proper bath for some time, and are used to a wash-down, and since they do not perspire, as do more active people, they are offended by the idea that they are dirty. Personal hygiene is subjective, and should not be imposed unless there is a very strong reason indeed, like overwhelming body odour, or sore skin. However, most people like to feel clean, and complain about too little care rather than too much.

It is worth noting that often it is very enjoyable to have a gentle brush-down with a dry, soft back brush before the complete wash-down. This gets rid of all the loose skin that can cause itching, and also encourages good circulation. It is well known as a beauty treatment but is also very enjoyable if you have the time.

CARE OF HEAD AND BODY HAIR

Hair is often a source of great frustration for both women and men. Some people find simply lifting their arms above their head so exhausting or painful that they need help before their carer expects them to.

Washing hair can be very difficult or even impossible for one person alone. Rubbing with a hot damp cloth or face flannel daily instead of a proper shampoo can help to lengthen the period between washing. There are dry shampoos available, but many people do not like using them and say they make the hair feel stiff.

It is worth looking around for other solutions. Sometimes local contacts can produce a reasonably priced home service. Sometimes a local charity will provide funding. Or friends will step in to help.

David found an ingenious solution. He was a taxi driver who over thirty years working locally had made many local contacts among his clients. He knew of a lady who had retired from hairdressing, and could not walk far because of her arthritis, and he arranged to collect her twice a week to wash and set his wife Lee's hair for a small fee. He might have had the same result from a local advertisement in the post office. Peggy was delighted to have a job, and the women became good friends. When it became more difficult to wash they obtained the loan of a useful tray from the local hospice, and the service continued for a year until Lee voluntarily had her hair cut, as she herself was tired of its length and heaviness. The new style was so easy to manage that her friend was still able to do her hair, though they were both less well and active by then.

Lee found a small bonus was that lack of housework meant her fingernails grew long and strong, as they had never done before. She transferred her interest in her hair to her hands, as they became soft and elegant with lack of use, and a great source of pride to her, as they were much admired. She loved having them painted, and her pre-teenage granddaughters were only too pleased to paint them for her, several times a day if she would let them.

Sometimes the only solution possible is not the one the patient would have chosen, but at least there is the knowledge that all avenues have been explored and considered.

Shaving is a necessity for most men, and even a beard needs attention if it is to look smart. For the man who prefers a wet shave, changing to the electric razor can be a difficult decision, but the electric razor is an easy solution if hands and arms are weaker, and if the carer is not a barber by trade. Wives are notoriously reluctant to take over the job of helping to shave someone, since it so often leads to arguments. However, sons and male friends can often step in and offer help, if the wet shave is the only acceptable practice.

Women also often shave their armpits and hate to have to ask for help with this personal detail. And for hair on any other part of the body, there is a veil of secrecy and embarrassment. Overcoming this takes time and sensitivity, but allowing facial hair to grow unchecked has a very detrimental effect on a woman's morale, which may be a little shaky anyway. There are many beauticians who will do treatments at home very reasonably, and again this is a very welcome gift when someone is unable to leave the house very often.

KEEPING A CLEAN MOUTH AND TEETH

It is very easy to forget to clean teeth when someone is in bed, feeling less than well a lot of the time. There is a current trend to offer a mouthwash instead of taking the time to clean teeth properly, and it is a poor alternative. If toothbrushes feel too large and result in a feeling of nausea, then often a child's toothbrush or an electric toothbrush is a solution. Even weak hands can manage an electric brush, and it can be very effective. There is no need to use a quantity of toothpaste, or indeed any at all if the taste is unpleasant, or spitting it out is a problem.

Cleaning another person's teeth is a difficult task, but using a damp brush and gently drawing the brush head away from the gum and up the tooth several times is neither difficult nor messy, and a much better option than rinsing out a mouth with mouthwash, several times a day.

If, over a period of neglect, the tongue becomes yellow and coated, there are several solutions. A very old-fashioned one is gently scrub the tongue with bicarbonate of soda solution, half a teaspoonful in half a cup of warm water. This may surprise people who have previously used it for cleaning ovens. For those who find oven cleaning a very satisfying chore, cleaning a mouth is equally rewarding! Sucking on a dispersible vitamin C tablet cleans tongues very well, and so does sucking chunks of pineapple. It is better to try to keep the tongue clean from the start, but so often it is not recognised as a potential problem until too late.

It is not always understood that there are dentists who will visit at home if someone cannot go to the practice. They can be of only limited help, but most hospices will have access to someone to help with a minor dental problem in such circumstances.

Mouths can sometimes develop an infection called thrush, which shows as white spots on the tongue, cheeks and throat. It can also cause a dry and 'furry'-sounding cough, and make swallowing difficult. It requires treatment with anti-fungal antibiotics, and is best dealt with immediately, as people find they lose appetite, and taste, and feel less well, if it continues. It also becomes more difficult to clear, with time. People who are debilitated because of illness or treatment, like radiotherapy or chemotherapy, are likely to develop thrush. It is something to keep a lookout for, so that it can be treated promptly by the doctor.

Keeping well hydrated is another way to ensure a mouth stays clean. Many people who are at home and bored do not want to drink, particularly if using the toilet is a lengthy and exhausting experience. Very few people drink a lot of water, so it is not a habit in the general population. However it is very beneficial for anyone, well or ill. Keeping a glass of water within reach encourages the practice, and many people find that regularly sipping water increases their thirst, and therefore their consumption. If water tastes horrible, either because of the locality, or because of certain drugs or treatment, then adding lemon juice or honey in tiny quantities can make it more palatable. Sometimes a fizzy drink like Coca-Cola is very cleansing. It is a question of finding out what is most acceptable. Try to average up to two litres of liquids a day, and see the difference it can make to your body, whether you are the carer or the patient. Also drinking a lot helps to keep bowels regular. This will be discussed later.

KEEPING RECORDS: ORGANISATION MAKES FOR EFFICIENCY

It is a good idea to make a plan of activities as they happen. This does not have to be complicated, and if started from day one will gradually develop, without being too time-consuming. Make it clear and succinct, and put it in a plastic cover. Then if new carers come in, there are clear instructions about what has to be done, and in which preferred order. A sample plan is shown on the next page.

The idea is that any visiting carer can also add to the chart, if they notice anything else that would be helpful to other carers.

It is also helpful if all the washing equipment is kept together and accessible, then there is no need for anyone to keep asking where the soap is and what cream is used, if any.

It is the same with medication. Keep it all together on a tray, or in a shoebox, with the list of times and the correct doses, then anyone stepping in as a carer has it all there on hand, and will not be asking questions all the time. Also, changes are easily recorded. An idea for a sample chart is shown below. The chart should be kept with the medication and placed in a plastic cover.

Some people use trays that can be bought for the purpose of preparing a week's medication, and this can be very useful if the medication is simple, or the patient or carer gets muddled with doses. However, having a proper chart means that anyone coming into the house can see immediately what needs to be given, and take responsibility for measuring out the doses. They can also identify any medication that can be given as an extra dose if necessary.

Sample Activity Plan

John Smith
DOB 11/3/1946
23 Some Street
London W3
Tel 0207 564 3321

John cannot speak very clearly due to his disease. However he is quite clear mentally and can indicate choices if they are clearly spelt out. He uses the electric toothbrush if it is held firmly for him, and he can move his head to position the brush. He likes his hair combed firmly, and parted on the left. He likes firm handling and feels insecure if you are too gentle. He needs to be encouraged to drink, as he is reluctant to increase his trips to the toilet. He can transfer easily from chair to bed etc. and will show you how to help him. He likes to have his face wiped dry first with a damp flannel, and please can you include his ears when you do this. If he requires the toilet he will make a T-T-T-T-T noise and that is the signal to get the toilet chair. On a good day he can walk there, and will shake his head and push on the arms of the chair to indicate this.

AM 8.00–8.15, breakfast
John likes a glass of water first with his medication, followed by cereal (in top right cupboard clearly marked) and served with warm milk and brown sugar. He likes a weak coffee with no sugar and plenty of milk, to finish.

AM 9.00 approx
John is taken to the bathroom in toilet chair, and will spend ten minutes on the loo. Please note if there is any bowel activity. He is then washed at the basin (his towels are all the blue ones, usually on the side of the bath). Fresh clothes are on the bath rail. He likes to have deodorant, but no talcum powder. All his toilet equipment is in a brown shoebox behind the door. He likes to have his hands, and feet too, gently scrubbed with the nailbrush if there is time. He likes his teeth cleaned last of all.

AM 10.00 approx
John will settle now in the garden room in his recliner chair. He has a fresh jug of water and glass on the table near to his left hand and a small bowl of chocolate and biscuits placed within reach, also the brass bell and the TV control. Once settled he has his medication put ready for 10.30 a.m. If anyone phones to suggest a visit he will confirm,

if not very clearly – and the time and day should be recorded in the red booklet.

PM 12.30, lunch
The tray with his lunch is on the top shelf of the fridge. If it needs heating please use the microwave. He needs a little help with handling cutlery. Please use the cloth provided to protect his clothes. If he wants tea he will write out a 'T' on the tabletop. He likes his tea quite strong and with a little sugar (half tsp). He likes some fruit cut up afterwards and will indicate his preference if shown some. He then goes to the toilet in his toilet chair, and from there to the bed for an hour's rest.

PM 4.30–5.00
He likes to go back to the sitting room, via the toilet, and have a cup of tea and some cake from the blue cake tin in the kitchen.

MEDICINE CHART SAMPLE

This is a sample chart unrelated to the John of the previous chart. It simply indicates the kind of information that would be useful to the reader, both as a reminder but also for the person who may be having to care for John unexpectedly.

Name	Time	Dose	Action	Comments
Morphine liquid 1 tsp	6.10 a.m. 6.10 p.m.	10 mg 2 tsp	To control pain	2 a.m. dose if awake
Morphine Tablets	Anytime in between other med	5 mg 1 tab	If in pain can have extra	If needed regularly please report
Diazepam Tablets	When needed	5 mg 1 tab	To calm if distressed	Can have 1 tab at night if required
Paracetamol	At any time	2 tabs	If there is bone pain	Not more than 8 tabs over 24 hours
Digoxin	9 a.m.	1 tab	To calm heart rate	

Chapter Nine

The Use of Aids and Appliances

Most people view the idea of having to accept an aid with apprehension and horror. It requires a degree of rethinking to view it as a welcome tool, enabling life to continue in as normal a way as is possible.

The story of Mary illustrates this view of an enabling tool very well.

Mary was an old lady living in the rural Midlands, just outside a small village. No one knew her exact age, but she had lived in her tiny cottage for many years. It had once been well out of the village, but as time passed the village became larger. When she began to find it very hard to return from her morning walk to the village shop, she managed to acquire a wheelchair (no one ever quite found out from where), which she pushed into the village every day. She did the shopping, and had a coffee, and then sat in her chair with her shopping on her lap and waited. Sure enough, someone soon stopped and asked if she needed help. And then found themselves pushing her the half-mile home. This obviously would not be advisable in central London, but it is her attitude that is interesting, rather than her solution to the problem. She simply saw the wheelchair as a positive asset to enable her to get around, rather than a handicap and a sign of giving in. So she set about using it as such.

That was not an easy attitude adjustment for her at eighty-plus years of age; it is much harder for someone younger.

Anna, aged seven, had a mother stricken with a neurological illness that left her struggling for every step she took. Anna was a very mature child, as she was the main carer during the day, while her dad was at work. Anna took a similar view of the situation, when she telephoned to ask a charity for the loan of a chair, '...for Mummy, because I am tired of having to help her walk in difficult places. When we went to the seaside one time I had to keep right by the car where she could see me. If she had a chair she could walk if she felt well enough, but if she didn't then Daddy could push her.' It took a little while to confirm the request and deliver the wheelchair, but after the first outing her mother admitted she had enjoyed herself for the first time in many months, The chair meant that she did not have to worry about return journeys when she was tired and weak. On a good day she could lean on the chair, and push it. When she became tired she retired to her chair, and allowed someone to push her.

If an aid can be regarded from the start as an asset to help keep someone independent, then it is much easier to accept the help it can provide.

Getting the Best Advice

Companies manufacturing aids to sell to the disabled have a vested interest in promoting their own equipment, though many are very ethical in their advice. Also, anyone trying to get financial help from Social Services for equipment, a difficult task at the best of times, will find it impossible if there has not been a professional assessment first.

Someone who has no knowledge of disability can be beguiled by advertisements, which appear to offer a solution to a problem. Someone who has experience of the illness, and the type of changes likely to occur, can see that a piece of equipment may only be of limited use, and for a short time. And indeed, no matter how useful a piece of equipment may be, no aid can ever truly replace a human limb. A constantly changing barrage of objects, all of which take up space and need instructions, and are then obsolete in a short space of time, when function has changed or lessened, can be depressing and demoralising at the very least.

Peter, who was in his sixties when his wife was diagnosed with a rapidly progressing form of multiple sclerosis, investigated every aid possible. He was an engineer, and felt he could decide for himself the most appropriate appliance, as he knew her needs on a day-to-day basis. The result was that over two years he spent a large part of his savings (about £17,000) on innumerable gadgets, many of which were of little if any use, as her condition changed so rapidly. Some helped for a few days; some were so complex that they were exhausting to use. Storage space was a problem and a whole room was devoted to storing all the gadgets.

After her death, he spent three years trying to empty the house of all the gadgetry. Unfortunately the second-hand resale value of such equipment is negligible. Even charities and Social Services are not able to accept them as gifts, because there is strict legislation regarding the loaning and maintenance of such equipment. Sometimes there is a response to private advertisements but there is still a heavy financial loss, not to mention the emotional stress of getting rid of all her equipment.

Expert advice is available through the local community services. Upon discharge from hospital, following a new diagnosis that has an associated disability, the family should be contacted by some of the specialists who may be able to help them. Before leaving the hospital it is always worth checking that one or other of the services have been requested by the hospital, and get a phone number so that you can make contact if there is any delay.

The occupational therapist, commonly called the 'OT', can advise on house adaptations and some equipment. Occupational therapists are also very clever at adapting and inventing ways of making disability more manageable. If some major changes are necessary, or it is felt that they may become necessary at some future time, the OT will also know the local financial limitations, and can help. The services an OT can offer can be limited at times, because of local policies and finances, and some OTs are hospital based, and will have to pass on a request to the community OT. They may also feel that a physiotherapist is better able to advise on, for example, wheelchairs, but for an initial contact the OT is the person to call.

For example, a shower is often the obvious choice for easy personal hygiene.

Many people do not have a shower, and will try to get one through Social Services. Success varies from area to area. However a shower can add value to a house, and is worth considering even if no grant is available. Sometimes a grant is possible, even if the person owns the house. Most aids are not a permanent feature, and it is possible in some circumstances to install a shower on temporary loan, from Social Services. Whatever seems to the family to be the best solution, an OT will have to make the initial assessment and referral to Social Services.

Sometimes it may be appropriate for a physiotherapist to be involved as well. The physiotherapist, often called the 'physio', will advise on physical symptoms like breathing freely, as well as keeping muscles flexible, and making best use of the patient's capabilities. Physiotherapists can offer advice on lifting and mobility, so that the carer is protected from damaging their own back, as well as perhaps hurting the patient.

Speech therapists and dieticians may be involved. This all seems an awful lot of strangers coming into the home, but many of them will not come regularly, and the ones who do can become valuable friends.

Inappropriate equipment is useless, and can be dangerous. People need instruction on using appliances, and monitoring to know when they are no longer appropriate.

All these specialists will also be able to offer support emotionally, depending on the individual. It is a good idea to accept their services, and to encourage them to give you as much information as they can.

Other Specialists Who Can Offer Ideas and Modifications

There are many excellent services available for the use of people who are trying to maintain their independence. Very often a very small adjustment can make a huge difference to the ability to remain an independent person. There are mobility-advice and vehicle-advice centres, often with a wide range of adaptations for sale, on loan or to hire. Anyone can ask for information from independent living centres, disability centres, mobility centres. A Citizens Advice Bureau will usually be able to give local advice, and a good community OT will know the sources of advice and help.

Laura, aged twenty-four and living in a rented flat alone, despaired because she could no longer give the correct foot pressure to change gear in her car, and an automatic gear change car was well beyond her means, unless she could continue to work. Her company were quite prepared to keep her employed for as long as she could do her job. She was popular at work and had run the company social outings for three years, so she was keen to keep her contacts. Her hands were also becoming slightly weaker.

Referral to the local mobility centre resulted in a simple adaptation, which served her well. They also helped her to apply for and receive financial help to buy another car with the correct adaptations, to enable her to continue driving. She was also thereafter under the care of the mobility centre, which gave her the security of continued monitoring, for the duration of her illness. The staff also became her friends, and another source of support. Sadly the day came when she could no longer drive, but she had the benefit of many mobile months, and continued contact with her young friends.

The OT can give information about mobility centres, and people can refer themselves. Anyone in similar circumstances to Laura is well advised to see if they can be helped in this kind of way. See the Appendix for further information.

Derek, aged forty-nine, had a very normal dread of becoming dependent on anyone for help with using the toilet. His anxiety was accentuated by his very sad marital relationship, so his wife would not help him with his personal care. A neighbour, who had happened to see information about a national exhibition for the disabled, gave him some information about help with using the toilet. With the aid of the OT assessment he felt more confident, and was able to maintain reasonable independence and privacy, for a great part of his illness. While nothing was a permanent solution to his problem, at least it helped for a while.

See the Appendix for helpful numbers for carers.

Chapter Ten

Some Common Symptoms and the Use of Medication

This chapter tries to give some awareness of how each individual can help themselves, to lessen common problems, and also gives a few general points to remember about medication. The best advice anyone can receive can be from the consultant with whom they have good rapport. Always try to find out if your consultant has a special interest in your disease. This is particularly true of neurological specialists, who often have to make difficult diagnoses from similar but slightly varying symptoms.

We have discussed physical comfort in Chapters Eight, Nine and Eleven, but it is worth repeating here that there are several aids on the market in the way of bedding, chairs and even beds and mattresses. Ask the district nurse, or the doctor. The experts are always the first line of information.

Exhaustion

Exhaustion is often an unexpected and disturbing symptom, and is more common than pain for many people. It can become the major day-to-day complaint of people with terminal illness, whether cancer or some neurological disease, or a chronic disease of heart or lungs.

It is important to remember that any activity uses up energy. Even talking to visitors is very tiring, especially when there is not a lot to say. Most people who are worried and apprehensive, ill and receiving treatment, or simply ill, have very little energy. No one who is well can understand or imagine the exhaustion that overcomes people with some common illness or disease. It is hard to imagine being terribly thirsty, and yet too tired to lift a glass of water. Too often a sick person is told to try harder, to make more of an effort, and sometimes the implication is that they are lazy.

Carers are often discouraged by what appears to them to be a lack of effort, and they nag and push in an attempt to make the sick person try harder.

No amount of nagging at someone can increase their energy. Understanding this and accepting the situation means that the carer can relax too, and respond to whatever energy levels the ill person is experiencing Allowing someone to take lots of catnaps, to snack whenever they please and to be as 'lazy' as they like eases a lot of tension.

Conserving Energy

Many people learn to conserve the energy they have. For example, if it is important to spend time with the grandchildren, and if the result of such an afternoon is the need to spend the following day quietly sleeping, then that is their choice and for them the result may be well worth it.

Conserving energy also applies to exercise, especially in many neurological diseases. People often feel that if they can use the weakening muscles, they can prevent further deterioration. In fact, excessive exercise, as when using exercise machines, can have the opposite effect and increase the weakness. This is particularly true with motor neurone disease, in the opinion of many specialists. It is not unusual for visiting professional carers to advise exercise in these circumstances, so the advice is always to ask the specialist and abide by their advice. Of course, as we have said, if there is a very strong reason for making a tremendous effort, then the usual advice is to go ahead!

Jeff was very anxious to see his only daughter graduate. He felt it would be worth the effort and the resulting tiredness, if he could just see her graduation. His determination was amazing, and with a team of helpers he was able to attend and have a light lunch beforehand with some of her friends. He then slept for nearly three days, and his carers claimed that they did as well. But it was worth it, and he was none the worse for the effort, when he finally woke up. It was a wonderful day for him, and for the whole family.

It also gave his morale and his confidence a huge boost.

Drinking Plenty of Water

As we have already said, drinking plenty of water helps to alleviate many symptoms, and is a vital part of taking care of oneself. Many nutritionists and osteopaths recommend two litres of water daily for healthy people, and many people who try it do notice an improvement in the way they feel. Even one litre of water daily can make a noticeable difference to the person who is ill. Drinking helps with constipation, especially drinking a glass of warm water on waking each day. Fluids also help prevent urinary infections, and help to maintain liver function, especially when on heavy medications. Most people having chemotherapy treatment are advised to drink plenty of water.

If there is always fresh water, perhaps with a touch of lemon juice or fruit juice by the bed or table, and the habit of drinking is embraced from the start, it is much easier to establish a good routine. And the person in bed will be less likely to have sore or dry skin. Commercially available drinks are often very sweet, and do not leave a pleasant taste, although, as we saw earlier, many people find Coca-Cola, tonic water or soda water leaves a clean feeling in the mouth.

There are of course many drinks available to help increase calorie intake. A pharmacist is able to give up-to-date advice, and it is also possible to have some of these on prescription in certain circumstances. It is important to remember that drinks left standing a long time become less appealing, and changing them is a chore easy to forget about, but which visitors are often grateful to perform. Some people suddenly find that taste changes, and they may enjoy herbal teas that were previously disliked. It is well worth trying an assortment of drinks that may have never seemed attractive before, like mint or cardamom tea. Both are made with ordinary tea or tea bags, with fresh mint or cardamom pods added to stand for a few moments.

Many Asian shops stock lovely varieties of tea that can appeal to people who have previously been happy with ordinary tea, and who now find that it tastes strange. A Thermos flask is useful to keep drinks cool or warm and thus more appetising, if someone is alone for long periods.

Of course, drinking more increases the number of trips to the toilet, and this can be very tiring. Keeping a urinal for a man, or a small bedpan for a woman, on a chair, covered with a clean towel, can help to reduce the time spent walking. It is possible to borrow a commode from the local authority, though many people resist this for as long as possible. It is possible to buy old ones in some second hand shops, which are quite well disguised as fairly comfortable chairs. Concerns about smell will be helped by regular emptying, keeping the pan absolutely spotless (another job for the carer) and by using a deodorant like Nil-Odour, which can be obtained from most chemists. The pharmacist is able to give very specific advice about this kind of problem, and is usually more than willing to share their expertise. If they are not helpful, then find another pharmacist.

Odours are a source of embarrassment to most people. Unfortunately, it is usually not effective to try to disguise an odour with another stronger odour. There are simple remedies, like striking a match or keeping a lit candle within range, or often a bowl of vinegar helps to keep a room fresh. High standards of hygiene and a constant source of fresh air is the most effective solution.

Sometimes it is hard for the patient to hold the glass or cup without help, which means another job for the carer. Eva's husband fitted up a long plastic straw pinned to the pillow and leading down to the glass. By simply turning her head she was able to drink when she felt like it without calling for help. Her intake of fluids increased greatly.

Two common results of immobility and illness, constipation and lack of muscle tone, can be lessened by early awareness on the part of the carer.

Constipation

Constipation is likely to affect everyone with a debilitating illness at some stage, and is often unrecognised until it becomes a major problem. Lack of exercise, reduced food intake, and often a reduction in dietary fibre, all add to the likelihood of someone developing constipation. Many painkillers cause some degree of constipation, and since this is a recognised side effect, laxatives should be prescribed with the drug and given from the start. When you are given a painkiller ask the doctor, 'Will this make me constipated?'

Many people are told that eating less will mean less output, and therefore to worry about missing a bowel movement daily is foolish. However, long ago, hospices identified constipation as a major problem among sick people, and the condition adds to the pain, discomfort, and indignity of any illness. Like a blocked drain, the large bowel slows down in its muscle function, and the blockage slowly builds up causing distension, headaches, colic, backache and nausea, as anyone who is occasionally afflicted will confirm. The remedy is to prevent the complication as far as possible. Any chemist will advise on a mild laxative to take regularly, before a problem develops. Many people will have a tried and tested solution that they have used during the times when they were well. Like a glass of red wine or beer, or certain fruit. Stronger painkillers or chronic constipation require strong laxatives, and sometimes a combination of medication, which acts in different ways on the bowel. Ask your doctor, and make sure he offers a solution.

Garry, aged thirty-three, had motor neurone disease, which although disabling, and often painful, did not make him feel ill. An enthusiastic beer drinker and sportsman, who had never experienced constipation, he listened to, but ignored the advice about his bowels – he had many other things on his mind as the disease progressed. At ten o'clock one evening he began to get severe abdominal pain, and strained to evacuate his bowels without effect. He became very distressed and agitated. Calls to the doctor resulted in advice to take the medication given to him, and the assurance that a nurse would call the following day.

He had a sleepless night, and so did the family. The nurse arrived late morning, but Garry required a doctor's examination before she could administer an enema. Garry was frustrated and angry and frightened and very tired. When he finally had the enema, it was insufficient to clear his bowels and the attempts continued for several days. It was undoubtedly the worst experience of his illness, and the most humiliating, and yet he had only been aware of the problem for a day.

Following the enema he started a regime of regular laxatives, increased fluids and fruit and vegetables, and the occasional suppository. Current laxatives can be combined and regulated to work well, without the sudden and explosive results that used to be dreaded by everyone, and which resulted in occasional incontinence.

Many people dislike taking any medication. It is true that all medication has side effects, and constipation is a common one. However it is more easily managed when it is treated early. People who are chronically constipated often complain of diarrhoea, because a chronic blocked bowel leads to a runny overflow. Often this is only cleared by several enemas. It is much better to watch out for it from the start, and to take the medication early on and continuously.

Loss of Muscle Tone

The second chronic condition that can be lessened through early awareness is loss of muscle tone and stiffness. This occurs as limbs contract due to muscle wastage, and lack of exercise. If someone is in bed for a while, the bedclothes can put pressure on their feet, making the feet drop and lose tone. Relieving the pressure, and encouraging regular movement of the feet, as well as supporting them with a very firm pillow or board, goes some way towards preventing a lot of discomfort and mobility problems later on. It is difficult to obtain physiotherapy at home in some areas. However it is usually possible to get advice and occasional supervision from a community physiotherapist to show the carer how to stretch, and give passive movements to unused limbs, to maintain some function.

It is very important to keep flexible. It need not take hours to learn how to perform simple exercises. Taking the time from the beginning saves time and pain later on. If there is a rehabilitation unit in the area, there is sometimes a possibility of accessing some care and advice from them.

Early awareness of the results of immobility can help to reduce the problem, or at least recognise it before it becomes chronic, and therefore more difficult to manage.

Obviously there are many symptoms that cannot be anticipated, and that have to be dealt with, as and when they appear. There is no point in scrutinising a sick person with a microscope all the time – that only leaves them feeling unsafe and apprehensive. General observation and a measure of common sense, and the ability to note a change and respond to it, are enough to keep a person comfortable, and hopefully avoid crisis.

Incontinence

Closely associated with these problems is incontinence. For many people the idea of becoming incontinent is the worst and most difficult part of any illness. In chronic situations there are surgical alternatives to consider, but initially there are no easy solutions.

One problem with incontinence is that the surrounding skin becomes extremely sore and can break down, and bedsores can develop very quickly indeed. There are many creams on the market but the real answer is prevention.

There are effective aids for male urinary incontinence, and a continence advisor can offer advice and suggestions. The very first step should be to attempt to use the toilet at very regular intervals. If this fails then some other method, or medical intervention is the next step. Often these aids are expensive, and expert advice on which to use is essential. For women the only answer is often the use of a catheter, which is a tube placed in the bladder, which can be free draining, or can be released at regular intervals. Long-term use of a catheter can cause problems and is generally not immediately advised by the doctor. All catheters need regular simple hygiene to prevent infection, but this is not difficult to learn to do. It is not a difficult procedure, and can be done at home. Again the advice is to ask the doctor or nurse. Get the answers you need, so that you understand the decisions being made, and are able to join in making them.

Incontinence of faeces is usually the most distressing symptom to manage. As we have said it is sometimes a side effect of constipation, as when the bowel becomes packed with hard stool, and the patient takes some laxative to soften the stool, which then bypasses the blockage, leading to the conclusion that the patient is now constipated, and incontinent. So if there is apparent diarrhoea, it is not always the time to stop laxatives. An examination by the doctor can establish the real situation.

Carers often assure the ill person that they do not mind at all cleaning them up after an 'accident'. This may be true, but it is not at all comforting to the person in the middle of the accident, who is degraded and humiliated by what has happened.

In truth, no one actually enjoys clearing up a soiled bed, whether they are family or professional carers. When the washing is to be done at home in the family washing machine, it is hard not to feel irritated and nauseated and if it happens frequently, harder to avoid showing it.

Once again, the advice is to resist the temptation to spray perfumes all around to cover up the odours, which do not help, and often irritate a cough or breathing difficulties.

Sometimes acknowledging the unpleasantness of the job is more honest, and yet again, recognising that the cause of the problem is not the person who is ill, but the illness itself, taking away all the dignity of the individual. Anger is less destructive if it is directed at the real source of the problem.

There are no easy answers. Again a good continence advisor can be a blessing, in helping to choose an effective appliance, or more often to advise on ways of timing the action of the bowels. Regular bowel action can sometimes be achieved with a combination of adequate liquids, medication and gentle abdominal massage. It takes a while to train the body but as long as constipation is not allowed to become a severe problem, it is possible to attain a level of bowel training, if not all the time, at least for the much of the time. (Abdominal massage can be as simple as gentle continuous pressure along the line of the large bowel performed after a warm drink early in the day. The gentle pressure should start at the right hand side of the abdomen, by the hipbone, and slowly move upwards to just below the ribs. Then continue the gentle pressure across the top of the abdomen, turning under the ribcage to pass down to the left hipbone.)

Understanding Medication

The quantity of pills prescribed is nearly always a source of concern and irritation. And, as we saw at the end of Chapter Eight, it is very useful at the very beginning to make a chart record of all pills, and the reason for taking them. Some people buy a pharmaceutical book, and study it carefully. This is not really necessary unless there is a special interest, but it is important to know why the pill is given, and when to take it. The pharmacist is often very helpful indeed in explaining everything, and it is well worth checking them out at an early stage. For people who want to know all the details, some information is available in the Appendix.

Gerry is a good example of the benefits of understanding medication. Gerry had been feeling very sick indeed following his chemotherapy. He was an accountant who worked on his own, and was not a talkative, let alone a complaining man. When he was actually sick, people paid attention, but since he rarely vomited and complained very little, no one seemed too concerned about his continuing nausea. However, he began to feel pretty fed up. He was nagged to eat and drink by his concerned family, as he became more lethargic and depressed. While in hospital he had been intermittently given an anti-sickness pill that had sent him off to sleep, and from which he woke up feeling better. When at home he took one, only when he was ill enough. In fact he was chasing the symptoms instead of anticipating them. After he was persuaded to take one pill at regular times, that is, on wakening and before each meal, he felt considerably better. Before long he was able to eat at regular intervals, and drink properly. He felt better able to cope with the ongoing treatment.

This also applies to pain medication. Marian had breast cancer for several years and managed well, until she was prescribed morphine. She was quite distraught, and very reluctant indeed to take it, as she thought this must be the last stage of her life. Finally, exhausted and upset, she accepted the explanation that it was the most effective method of pain control, and she began to take a very small dose indeed at regular four-hourly intervals. She was given a small dose of anti-sickness medication to match the morphine as it sometimes causes nausea, and for the first day or two she was a little sleepy. However two days later she began to feel so much better that she was actually planning outings, and thinking about what to eat for lunch. Once home she was able to continue her role as mother and wife, in much the same way as before, and as her mood was happier, so the family also felt happier.

Steve was only in his twenties. He was an athletic man, newly married when he was diagnosed with a rare form of cancer of the chest. He was strongly motivated to stay active for long enough to try and ensure a safe financial future for his new young wife, so he took a great interest in all the process of his illness. He was especially interested when he was offered morphine to control his severe pain, because he had always been opposed to any form of drugs.

Once out of pain, he read up all he could about the medication, and was soon able to explain it to all his visitors. He was able to continue to drive his car short distances very safely, to go to the cinema, entertain friends, drink his favourite wine and generally lead a fairly normal life. He regulated his dose himself, which he was encouraged to do, as it was given in liquid form every four hours. He remained pain-free for the rest of his illness, often reducing his morphine for days at a time. He felt in control of his medication, and was very responsible about the use of the drug.

The secret of successful medication is to be ahead of the symptoms and not chasing them. Waiting until the pain is severe before taking something means that the pain never completely goes, and the patient is always waiting for it to return. The same situation happens with nausea or vomiting. Dealing with the symptom before it becomes a problem is better than chasing it when it has become one, and has created anxiety, which in turn heightens the awareness of the unpleasant symptom.

Many people fear that if they take too much medication they will become used to it, and will no longer benefit from it. This is a fallacy. There are specialist symptom-management units attached to many hospitals and hospices. If a GP is not specialised, and seems nervous of increasing medication, then it is well to ask for a referral to a specialist unit. There is absolutely no need to suffer unnecessarily.

Many people also use homeopathic advice, and this can be very effective indeed in spite of the fact that the art has never been fully proven. However, for the patient, a certificate to prove the pill works is not as important as feeling relief from an unwelcome symptom, and many people with a strong antipathy to medication have found this to be a very helpful alternative. A classical homeopath will only suggest one remedy at a time, and will work in conjunction with the medical treatment already prescribed. Again the pharmacist in a homeopathic pharmacy is usually knowledgeable, and happy to help with advice.

'Healing' has also been found to be useful by some people, though also not proven. However, do not be discouraged by negative responses, because if something helps at all then it has to be a bonus. Complementary therapies can be found listed in your Yellow Pages directory.

Many people believe prayer to be very helpful, no matter to whom or to what deity the prayer is directed. Again this is a matter of personal choice. How much it helps is what is important, and at least there are no nasty side effects to these remedies

Chapter Eleven

Physical Comfort, Health, and Safety for Everyone Involved

Clothing

Clothing is an important part of our body image. We may wear a suit or a uniform or a tracksuit, but whatever we wear puts us in a category that others identify. It also reinforces our own view of ourselves. Even the most casually dressed person is making a statement. When the choice of what to wear is taken away we feel undermined and there is a huge loss of confidence. A man suddenly unable to wear a suit because he can no longer button his shirt and zip his trousers and tie his tie, feels a lesser person and has to make some huge adjustments to the way he sees himself.

Someone who has never worn a tracksuit strongly resists the idea when it is forced upon him. It is much easier if a person has some control over when to change the way they dress. To look for alternatives at the first sign of difficulty is to take an easier approach. There are many ideas to help with dressing and clothing problems, and information is available at any of the specialist units around the community, and in hospitals. Any organisation or charity that relates to disability can give specific advice or direct the question to someone who can help.

For a start, it is easy to replace zips and hooks with Velcro, which is undetectable from the outside and very easy to do without a degree in sewing. Women sometimes find it easier than men to adapt to a change of clothing since there is more variety in women's clothing. Items like pop sox are a wonderful aid to getting dressed without too much effort.

Again, clothing can be a problem for the carer, who needs to be comfortable as well as feeling able to go out and shop, in between nursing the patient. Few people can easily replace a complete wardrobe, but as clothes are replaced there is often a clear indication of how the situation is developing. Almost always there is an early necessity for low-heeled and practical shoes, at least around the house.

Lifting and Moving Someone Safely

Lifting someone who is weak and less mobile, without injuring either person, requires some practice. Enthusiastic carers can damage themselves without realising it, only to discover that another legacy of the illness is lifelong back pain. Professionals are restricted in the weights they are legally allowed to handle, currently a total of five stone between two people. Unfortunately, there is no protection for the carer at home, and the average adult weighs considerably more than five stone, and may very well maintain a higher weight throughout the illness. Useless limbs are surprisingly heavy.

Because of this regulation about lifting for professionals, if there is a likelihood of immobility, a hoist is immediately placed into the home by Social Services. It is very sensible to learn how to use this, even though there seems to be no need for it in the near future. Meantime, there are ways of helping to move someone without causing him or her too much discomfort.

For example if the patient can tolerate wearing a thick belt, the carer can grip it and lift without pulling on arms and shoulders.

People with neurological diseases often have weak arms and shoulders, and therefore cannot offer resistance when they are pulled. People who have had, or are undergoing radiation or surgery in the upper body, also can become very weak. Even though the limb may appear quite normal, tugging at the shoulder may result in acute pain and muscle damage. A physiotherapist will often be able to offer advice, and sometimes the district nurse (if there is one involved) can loan a lifting tray, similar in principle to a thick belt. There are several aids, and it is very wise to search around for any method of protecting both carer and patient. Avoid underarm lifting, which is extremely uncomfortable at best, and at worst painful, for the person who is being moved, and should never be used (though it can still be seen to be applied in some hospitals).

Carers must consider themselves when trying to lift the person who is ill. Living with a back problem can be a lifelong reminder of a period of illness, which will never be forgotten anyway. It is very important to avoid injury, and since there is often little understanding among the professionals of the role of the carer, it becomes the responsibility of the owner of the back. Also, having a bad back makes life generally very difficult. Sometimes families find their own solution with unorthodox and unrecognised gadgets. A good physiotherapist will advise on safety issues and offer suggestions.

Eating and Taking Nourishment

Meals are often a source of stress to the carer when there seems so much to do in so little time. Again, food is of equal interest to both carer and patient. It is easy nowadays to have access to ready prepared meals, but these are often high in fat and very expensive.

It is all too easy for the carer, while concentrating on the person who is ill, to neglect their own needs, eating only snacks and leftovers. This results in the carer putting on, or losing weight, and suffering a loss of energy and general debilitation. This can be a source of concern to the observers, one of whom may well be the person who is ill.

Here are some ideas for healthy eating:

Homemade soups are quick to make, easily digestible and very nutritious as well as being fairly cheap. All that is needed is a liquidiser, and very often a charity will provide this, if finances are a problem. A few bones and a pile of vegetables easily make up into nourishing and tasty soup.

Fresh fruit is very filling and healthy, and people with small appetites can enjoy quality ice cream, or homemade custards, or yoghurts. Cheese can end a meal if the carer has had very little of the main meal. Often friends are glad to help out with the occasional meal, especially if they know how much the gesture can help.

Making milkshakes is quick and they are very nutritious, especially when honey, cream, ice cream or food supplements are added to the mixture.

As mentioned earlier, there are many food supplements on the market, which are designed for persons unable to take in adequate nourishment, for a variety of reasons. Some of these are quite pleasant and can be enjoyed, but it is still very much more sociable to be able to sit and eat proper food, if possible. A pharmacist can offer advice on food supplements, and it may be possible to acquire some samples. Some are available on prescription.

Elsie, aged seventy, had always had a small appetite when she was well, but was given several tins of food supplement to drink per day, most of which she disliked and found too heavy. Mealtimes could have become a battleground, but Alan, a keen amateur cook, preferred to add glucose, eggs, cream, high-calorie ice cream or honey to her normal food. The only problem was that his weight matched, and eventually overtook hers. He encouraged her to have small frequent drinks of the supplements in between his homemade meals, and he enhanced their taste with honey and occasionally alcohol. They never used the whole supply, but she maintained a satisfactory weight for her condition, and enjoyed her food.

Any dietician from a hospital will be glad to offer advice and suggestions to people who find tinned food unattractive. A glass of wine or sherry will go happily alongside most medication – the doctor will usually confirm this – and again a bottle of wine is a nice and not too expensive gift for anyone to buy.

Carers need to care for themselves with the same affection as they do the sick person. Little treats are important, and most sick people are always anxious about the person who looks after them, and are glad to see them well cared for as well.

Peter's wife (mentioned earlier in Chapter Nine) regularly treated herself to a trip to the hairdresser and came in to tell him, 'There's another £20 off your payslip this month' (actually his benefit allowance), and he was always delighted, and far more appreciative of her appearance than he had been in happier times.

Losing Weight

It is easy to become fixed upon the idea of not losing weight, and this is often encouraged by the hospital on outpatient assessments. However, a large proportion of people who are ill and immobile will eventually lose weight. And this can cause great anxiety. In fact the few who actually increase their weight may find that they appear flabby and fatty and the weight gain does not make them look healthy. Also very heavy people are more difficult to care for, and often develop sore skin and bedsores. (Weight gain can be a big problem, and is often seen in people with cerebral tumours and people who have to take high doses of steroids for a long time to help with symptoms.)

However if there *is* weight loss the carer begins to feel a failure, and will nag the patient to eat, often making mealtimes miserable. It is sometimes better to take the attitude of encouraging food in small and frequent quantities, enjoying what is eaten, and leaving the hospital to worry about the weight. (In fact, many hospital and most hospices no longer get concerned about weight loss, but they do not always seek to reassure the family, so they do not worry either.) Small tasty snacks, 'grazed' over several hours, can be much more enjoyable when someone is not hungry, and just appreciates a treat to relieve the boredom.

Changes in Sense of Taste

It is also a fact that not just the disease, but also certain treatments can cause a change in the taste buds of some people. Radiation and chemotherapy are the common culprits, and complaints of too much or too little salt, too much or too little sugar, frequently follow these treatments. Sometimes taste can change for no apparent reason. This can lead to a lot of family disagreements, so if there is some understanding of the problem there is less likelihood of many serious misunderstandings. It is also fairly common for a person to dislike the texture and flavour of meat. It is better to accept these changes and modify a diet than to try and force unwanted food onto an unwilling patient.

Sitting Comfortably

If a person is spending a great deal of time sitting they inevitably become very stiff and aching. If they have lost weight as well they become very sore quickly, and skin sores can develop, especially when they are wriggling around trying to ease an ache. It may be better to have a variety of chairs within reach to move to, and thus change position slightly. Altering pillow arrangements can also alter pressure. Having plenty of pillows to hand makes it much easier to achieve a level of comfort. An armchair arrangement, like placing pillows in an armchair or triangular shape, is an effective way to support a person in bed, or in a chair.

There are also various ways of protecting skin, like sheepskin covers for chairs, and inflatable cushions. Again it is worth trying whatever is offered. Foam or air-filled rubber rings were the only option at one time, but these are no longer used within the health service, and are in fact actively discouraged, though many people find them very useful, for short periods of time only. Almost all of them can be borrowed from the local authorities after an assessment by the physiotherapist or OT, or bought fairly cheaply from a chemist. Ask the district nurse, or one of the visiting specialists for advice. Likewise there are beds and mattresses available on loan if there is a need, and if the specialists feel they will benefit the patient, and the carer. Sometimes you need to ask them.

It is not unusual for someone to be unwilling to have a different bed in the home, and this is entirely understandable. However, if it can be made nearly as comfortable as your own bed, and it means that the care given can be much improved, because the person in the bed is more accessible, and easier to lift, then the benefits must be weighed and considered.

One way to help is to change position as often as is possible, and thus relieve the continuous pressure on back, and spine, and buttocks. A way to do this is by using an electric riser recliner chair, which is available from social services in many areas, or with some illnesses can be provided on long loan by a charity.

The riser recliner chair is also very useful indeed if someone has trouble pulling themselves into an upright position. It saves a lot of energy and so enables someone to walk a short distance, which perhaps they could not do if they had to exhaust themselves getting up. Again, to ensure the chair is really supportive and comfortable, the patient needs to be measured to make sure that the length of their thighs, for example, is right for the depth of the chair seat. And consideration of the patient's leg length is important so that the chair is not too high, and also to ensure that their legs are well supported, and do not just hang down.

A slight change of position makes a lot of difference. It is not necessary to move to another chair to achieve this, and again a good physiotherapist can advise. It is very comforting, though now no longer considered necessary, to have the area under pressure gently rubbed with a nourishing cream at intervals, and especially in the morning when getting up, and at night when going to bed.

Carers too should have comfortable chairs and beds. Chrissie slept for so long on a Z-bed by her husband that she developed chronic back pain, which blighted her life for five years following his death. Many people perch on the edge of the bed for long periods over many weeks and then suffer from the physical effects.

Individual Suggestions for Specific Problems

With some illnesses the neck muscles become very weak, and holding their head up can be too much effort for the sick person. There is a variety of supports, but very often a bandanna tied around the forehead and crossing over loosely to include the back of a high chair is a temporary and effective solution. It may not look comfortable to the observer but many patients find it an excellent solution. Again a physiotherapist can help with this problem. It is well worth contacting a charity that relates to specific diseases, to ask advice on specific problems. Many people feel an understandable reluctance to attach a label to themselves, when they feel they have lost enough individuality, but these charities do have a lot to offer, and do not usually intrude beyond answering questions, and offering support.

Understandably, there is some resistance to moving furniture around a settled home, and the changes can only emphasise the transition from healthy person to invalid. Small changes are easier to arrange. Loose rugs are a hazard if walking is difficult. Small pieces of furniture can become obstacles. Lighting may need adapting. These small changes are easier to accommodate and can make a big difference. If there is a nice view from one point then rearranging the room so that the view can be appreciated as much as possible is an obvious change.

As time passes it may be that bigger changes are necessary, and if they take place as part of a long ongoing process, they are easier to accept.

Unfortunately, some extra equipment is often needed, and if it has to be regularly used it can become the focal point of a small room. This problem has to be managed – it can be very hard, if not impossible, to prevent the room looking like a hospital extension. Often an outside visitor can see a way to hide the evidence, which is such a reminder of sickness.

Sometimes a local support group has relevant experience and can be a great help and support and offer original suggestions. The best solution: welcome suggestions, but take time to think them over, and do not be harassed into major changes made in a hurry.

Chapter Twelve

Children: Managing Change and Planning for the Future

With all the changes in their environment, what particular needs do the children in such a family have? Children adapt quite well if the changes accommodate their requirements to a degree. As discussed in Chapter Five, they can become very difficult if they are anxious, and they have unanswered questions. That is not to say they have to know all the details, but even very small children will become aware of unhappy atmospheres, and will often overreact and become the focus of attention, as they try to distract the family from the problems.

Unless they have had a very regimented existence previously, children will adapt to changes in their routine, if they take place gradually. Mealtimes can be varied slightly, and if the food prepared is nourishing for an adult, it is certainly nourishing for a child. They often miss the type of contact they used to have with the person who has become ill – the games, the physical activities – especially if the father is the sick parent. Small children cannot understand why they cannot indulge in the rough playing that fathers do so well. Sometimes a male relative can take over some of their role, but it is painful for a parent to watch this happening.

Charlie, aged thirty-one, was too weak to play with his son of three as he had done only a few months previously, and before he developed motor neurone disease. He had been a keen amateur footballer, but his wife was a tiny fragile woman, who was quite unable to engage in rough play with the little boy. He had a cousin who offered to visit on a regular basis each week, to play rough and tumble with the little boy, in the family home, under Charlie's watchful eye. The cousin had two small daughters, and enjoyed the different aspects of play with a small boy.

There are obvious potential problems with this kind of situation, but in this case it worked well without the child transferring his affections, and without the small girls becoming jealous. The three children became quite close, almost like siblings. The regular playtimes gave the family a break, and when he was at home with Charlie the small boy found quieter ways of amusing himself. When Charlie was given a blanket with swirling colours on it the child found he could make roadways in the pattern, and he spent many hours driving his toy cars gently over the ruts and patterns in the blanket, with some accompanying noises, giving his father ample time to observe him with great amusement.

Several years after Charlie died the two families were still close, with the children continuing to behave very much as siblings, though Charlie's widow had remarried and was expecting a new baby.

Allowing Children to Help

Alan and Betty had children who were old enough to help, and were very proud to be trusted with jobs like helping Daddy at mealtimes, getting him a warm damp cloth to wipe his hands, or rubbing his hands with cream. Far from becoming careworn little carers, it seemed that they took pride in their 'jobs', and having given the help they were ready to dash off to a friend's house and play. Also, they had room enough in their own home to invite friends in for television and playing house, so perhaps they felt that things had not changed too much.

If people are honest with the children as far as they are able, the children will learn to accept explanations, and feel secure in the knowledge that they will not be lied to. They can therefore lead relatively normal lives, and trust their parents to keep them up to date with the situation. In the event of the death of the parent, they have a legacy of trust that will be a support to them for the rest of their lives.

It is very hard not to lean too heavily on the child for support, and that is why it is always a good idea to encourage other people to be aware of the situation. This means the child or young person can confide in someone outside the family if they need to, without feeling that they are breaking confidence and telling family secrets. It is also good for every member of the family to allocate, or have allocated, some time in which they can relax and recharge their emotional and physical batteries.

When Parents Cannot Agree

The other important point to remember with children is that sometimes parents do not agree when they are trying to protect each other from noise or interruption. Ruth had four children, she came from a large noisy family, and she had never worked outside the home. She was an easygoing and relaxed mother, who worked around the needs of her growing family. Matthew, her husband, had been an only child, and was a workaholic who was usually only home in time for goodnight kisses all round. He found the children's noise and disorder very distracting.

When he became a part-time carer with live-in paid help, he immediately arranged the children's day so that they were rarely at home, and he could work in peace. Ruth became more silent and withdrawn, and it was the children's grandmother who eventually discovered that she was missing the noise and laughter that was normal in her house. She had tried to be as little trouble to Matthew as possible, and she also thought it would upset the children if they always saw her in bed, and as a result she was losing her family as well as her health.

It took some negotiation to ensure that Matthew could work in peace in his corner, while Ruth settled happily with the accustomed chaos around her. The children soon became used to the idea that she was in bed in the middle of everything, and at times took advantage of her lack of mobility, and had to be gently disciplined by their father.

They did not seem concerned by Ruth's gradual deterioration. It was just part of life. If the noise became too much for her on some days, it was not so different from a normal mother getting irritated and shooing the children to another house to play.

Accommodating children has to be flexible, and for some mothers the noise and the distraction of the family when they are ill may prove too much for them. Sharon had five children, and had also always had part-time work. When she developed a brain tumour, she tried to plan a timetable to cater for the children in the way she could manage best. She had them in rotation for an hour one day, or two hours another day, and friends filled in for her with the help of the school. She simply could not manage more than one child at a time.

Differing Opinions on Helpful Appliances

Patrick, always a loud and boisterous communicator, became unable to swallow or speak clearly, due to his neurological illness. He found that he was frustrated and angry because the children ignored him. While his wife, Beth, was able to understand him, he was reluctant to borrow any aid, and relied on her to interpret for him. His speech and language therapist took a long time to persuade him, but eventually he borrowed a lightwriter. This is a battery-operated machine for writing out messages, which were then reproduced in a dalek-type voice with an American accent. Patrick hated it on sight, but soon found that the children responded well and quickly as he relaxed, and became confident in using it. The children showed it to everyone, and surprisingly began to learn to spell with it. Even his four-year-old could understand small words that were commonly used, and she talked back at the machine very confidently, to the extent that she would cover the screen with her chubby fingers and say, 'Wait a minute, Daddy, I'm talking.'

These machines are constantly improving in design. Again the speech and language therapist, commonly known as SALT, will also be the person to consult if there are problems with swallowing. It is important to emphasise that no one has to be computer literate to adapt to these machines, they are designed for all abilities.

(Just a reminder here that the speech and language therapist will also be the person to advise if there are problems swallowing, so he or she is invaluable in any neurological disease and should be involved from the beginning.)

Sadly, as a general rule, the illness progresses and ideal solutions have a way of becoming obsolete, but if something can be provided that works really well for a short time, does not take up a lot of room, and is not prohibitively expensive, it is a bonus.

Getting Support in the Early Days Following Diagnosis

Some people have found that a course of massage, or regular talking time with a local volunteer support group, has provided space to gain perspective and support, especially during the early days of a diagnosis.

Richard had early support from his local OT, who arranged for his three children to be taken to a summer school nearby, to give the family a much-needed break, when he received his diagnosis at the beginning of the summer holidays.

Vera had her small baby looked after in a crèche run by Social Services, for just two afternoons a week throughout her illness, which gave her the time she badly needed to rest. She was able to specify the most convenient times for her.

For parents used to being the carer, and the one in charge, it is very hard indeed to relinquish that role. However, as new parents have to learn to leave their babies in nursery, or with friends, so the sick parent will find it easier to allow others to help with their children as time goes by, especially when they can see the benefit to the child. All young people need to be able to escape from the sickroom sometimes, and to have fun and laugh with friends without feeling guilty. In the early days of the diagnosis, it is very necessary to move away a little at times, to help gain some perspective on what is happening. No person can remain in crisis indefinitely, whether physical or emotional. Without relief, there will be a breaking point of some sort eventually.

Planning for the Future

Many people plan in a detailed way for the day when they will no longer be there for their children, leaving memory boxes, or writing books and letters. Some cannot think of such a sad loss, and prefer to act as if nothing will ever change. There is no one way that has the absolute answer for everyone.

There are many examples of people doing remarkable things in the last few months of life, parents preparing their children for the time when they will not be around for them. Some people set up charities for research, or for new equipment for the local hospital, people climb mountains and run marathons. They are to be admired, but there are also many thousands of ordinary people who leave behind them wonderful legacies for those closest to them.

Grace, aged forty, left a scrapbook behind for her three young children, lovingly built by her over the course of her three-year illness. An older parent, she had been a great career woman, and had many entertaining stories about her work abroad in education. The book also contained thoughts about the children's future, lots of stories about her childhood and her children's babyhood. She put funny stories in on small scraps of paper about her courtship with Tim and how they met. She wrote about the children starting school, and some of their holidays they had enjoyed. She had pleasure from making it, and was glad to think that they would have pleasure reading it. It also gave them a history of their mother, and she hoped it would influence them in choosing a career, when the time came.

Anne, who ran a pub with her husband Mick, bought Christmas presents early for her two children, and her parents and husband. They all co-operated in the planning and scheming for the others, not knowing that the surprise included them too. The presents were all lovingly labelled, and retrieved from the wardrobes around the house after her death. Her son, aged six, was asked by her: 'I want you to plan a very special Christmas present for this year, just in case I can't buy something special for you again. So this is a very important present and I want you to think about it very carefully because it must be something you will always love, not just a car or a bike.'

His reply amused the whole family when he said, 'I know just what I want. It's one of those small cards that they advertise on TV. You can just pay for anything with it and it lasts for years.' He paused and added, 'I think there are ones with a blue pattern in the corner as well, and they are just as good.'

He had grown up with his parents paying bills as goods were delivered, and was very aware of the existence of credit cards.

Patrick, mentioned earlier, realising that his voice was fast vanishing, went down to the local funeral directors and paid for his funeral, sorting out all the general arrangements, but leaving enough flexibility for Beth to have her say, if she wanted to. She realised what he had done only after he died, and she could appreciate what a generous gift he had left for her, in relieving her of all the stress of arranging and paying for his funeral.

There is a group called the Rosetta Life Project (see Appendix), which assists people in making a video or tape as a record of their life for their children, so that they feel the children will remember them, and know them a little, especially if the family are young. Many amateurs have managed to do this for themselves with family help.

People do what they feel they can do, and what is appropriate for them and their family. Whatever they do gives them satisfaction, and is done with love, and accepted with gratitude. There is sometimes almost subtle pressure to make huge impacts on the outside world, but this is not the tactic for most people. It is enough for them to manage their illness, and to know that they have done their best.

What to Say About Dying

One thing that always concerns people is what to tell a child about dying. Again this is very personal depending on the belief of the family. Some children get a lot of comfort if they think their parent or sibling is a star looking down on them forever. Some find the idea distressing and a bit frightening. Some children, when told that God wanted Mummy so badly that he took her away from a small child who also wanted her badly, can only imagine a very mean and cruel deity. Others feel that their mummy was a very special person to be so needed. One small girl had been told that her granny had gone to a beautiful place where everyone was happy and no one was ever sad, and she wanted very much to join her, and felt even more that she was 'not good enough'. Yet another believed she would go to Devon to meet her mum again, having misheard the word heaven.

Death at any age is a huge change and loss, and most people feel inadequate in trying to support young children through such a trauma. Perhaps if you have no strong beliefs the best way to approach this is to tell the child honestly what you believe. If you truly believe that you are going to heaven you can convince the child. If it is just a trite saying, the child will recognise the insincerity. Most children can understand that sometimes things happen that no one can explain, however clever they are, and we have to live with not understanding. All children know that bad things happen to some very nice people, and nice things happen to bad people too. They may be very fearful of losing other people whom they love. All we can do is to try and ensure that the experience does not leave them too fearful and apprehensive of the future.

Chapter Thirteen

Long-term Care: Unhappy Families and Mental Health

It is rarely possible to anticipate accurately the length of time that someone may be ill or incapacitated, and, whether the prognosis is long or short, most people have in the back of their minds the question of how long they really have to live. If the illness or disease progresses at a calm and peaceful rate, the idea of long-term illness becomes more familiar, though not necessarily less frightening or more acceptable.

After the initial shock of diagnosis, and the strain of adapting to changed and changing routines in the home, life often settles into a pattern set by a lot of outside influences. The initial expectation of an early death may mean the patient has done a lot of planning and arranging, and when death does not come as expected, there is a feeling almost of irritation and lack of motivation, and of being let down by the experts. There is also a feeling that everything has been tidied up and finished, and the patient at the centre of the situation is almost redundant.

One of the hardest aspects of accepting disability is accepting the change in role that accompanies health changes. It is hard to remain an onlooker as other people take over one's own role of father, mother, breadwinner, cook, housewife, however much they may have wished to change their role at times. It is pointless offering activities that are of no relative value, and that are recognised as pacifying and filling time. To remain part of the family a person has to believe he or she is contributing. This can happen when the sick person is so beloved that they remain the focal point of the whole unit, just by being there. This can happen naturally with people who are well, as age gradually causes them to relinquish their role in the family. For someone who suddenly becomes ill, it is more difficult. Most people have a need to fulfil a function that can be identified and quantified.

Being Appreciative is Not Always Easy

This means that there has to be appreciation on both sides. Saying thank you has a gratifying effect on both parties, and being appreciated encourages everyone to make further efforts.

With many long-term illnesses, the day-to-day symptoms are not acute and very often a person will show small changes over a longish period. Of course, at times acute symptoms can occur such as breathing difficulties, or vomiting or sudden pain. Some of these changes, if not so much expected, can to an extent be anticipated. That is why monitoring by the professional team is so valuable, and means that treatment can be offered immediately. Treatments like radiotherapy or chemotherapy may also cause a sudden change, but this often soon resolves and life continues as usual.

Neurological disease is less predictable, and there may be sudden and unexpected change, depending on the disease. Therefore it may be helpful to get as clear a picture as possible of what *can* be or *might* be expected. Often the really useful information comes from a special interest group or charity, because they will probably have compiled comprehensive information that covers all eventualities.

Misdiagnosis

There is sometimes a high rate of misdiagnosis among some neurological diseases. There are also many newly identified diseases, about which less is known, and so the progression of some neurological illnesses can be uncertain, and the family can feel very bewildered. At the beginning, the patient wants the diagnosis to be anything but what he has been told. Life can become a search for a solution, for a better diagnosis or different treatment, or for another opinion. Yet, if after some time, when plans have been made, a person is told that all has changed, this can be as upsetting as the initial diagnosis. The original label is the patient's identification, and he or she has often become an expert in this disease. Their expertise is taken away as well as their identity, and often their future expectations become even more uncertain.

Looking for Another Role in the Family

After a short time in bed or immobile, there is very little to talk about since every day is much the same. The initial drama and grief and fear of imminent loss have receded, and the inactive or ill person can gradually become less connected to the family unit, and less involved in family activities. It is easy for the sickroom to feel remote and isolated, and the person who lives there to become distant and more self-centred. For them, it begins to feel as if there is no other life outside that room. The one who is not ill, the carer, has to bear the brunt of most decisions, as well as the general running of the house, and so communication can be less open.

However, it does not have to be like this. With honesty and trust the emphasis may change, but both partners can find a meaningful role in the life of the family.

Alec, aged fifty-seven, was always very much the man of the family, working hard, managing the finances, and coming home daily to find his meal waiting for him, and the household chores completed. When he fell ill with a disabling form of spinal cancer, he was unable to appreciate that Ellen had to start to work to help finances. She had never needed to work. Now she worked as a school dinner lady, did child-minding for two thirteen-year-olds who lived next door, as well as ironing for her neighbours, and any other menial work that helped her to pay her way. Alec could not bear to see her work in such a way, and sitting in his chair he issued orders, and opinions, and suggestions, which did nothing to boost her confidence, nor show any appreciation of her efforts to keep the family together. They were fast reaching a stalemate situation where they felt they could no longer live together, however ill he became, when they finally asked for professional help.

Alec tried to view the cancer as an uninvited outsider who had nothing to do with him, but was an intruder within the family. Once Alec began to appreciate that Ellen was maintaining the family in the only way she could, he began to value her courage in a more detached way, and to feel less as if he were to blame. He then began to help a little by taking over the child-minding part of her day, by talking to the children and playing cards with them, an activity they loved, and which taught them a great deal. As he focussed more on what he could do to help Ellen, he began to take an interest in the meals, and even plan the menus as far as making a shopping list. Ellen found this very useful since she could never think of what to eat, though she was happy to do the cooking as usual. As he became less angry and bitter, they relaxed more together and began to chat and communicate in the way they had been able to when he was well.

There were many days when he felt the despair and frustration return, but he never lapsed completely into his initial emotional state. Ellen felt she could cope with anything but the anger, criticism and negativity she had first encountered with him. Although he did become very weak, he was able to play a very rich role in the life of the family, and so began to cope with his illness with great dignity. He also took over the financial planning and budget of the house, and set up ways to make it easier for Ellen to take over, when he was no longer there.

As illness progresses and people adjust to the many changes, the speed of change may appear to slow down. If this does happen, there is time for the family to think through the experience, and feel more in control of daily events. However, often there are still frequent changes in the type of help, and the numbers of helpers. Professional carers come in at times to suit the needs of a number of clients, rather than an individual. Understandably, most people prefer an early-morning visit so they can then have their day free. However that choice is rare, as the professional carer can only plan visits in the order of distance travelled, how long each visit can take, and the needs of the client. Others will have to wait their turn. Over time people can begin to feel quite institutionalised, even in their own homes. It takes effort and imagination to resist this. Carers also change frequently, and favourites move on, and new people come, and have to be told what to do and how to do it. Equipment is brought in, used, and then removed, as it becomes ineffective. It is easy to lose heart and become depressed and impatient, and make little effort to help in whatever ways may be appropriate.

As we said before there has to be appreciation and encouragement on both sides. Saying thank you has a gratifying effect on both parties, and being appreciated encourages everyone to make further efforts.

How Can Unhappy Families Cope?

Not all families are happy and close before illness strikes. There are some families and groups who have long grown apart, and will never be able to forge bonds again. This is a situation that has to be accepted also, and it may be that what seemed like an inevitable break-up will become a reality far more quickly in the face of this kind of illness.

Margaret and John, both in their mid-forties, with no children and strong separate careers in the business world, were on the verge of divorce when he was diagnosed with cancer. He underwent all the investigations alone, while she continued to work, and to make plans to leave him at some time. When he received his final diagnosis, she felt absolutely trapped and bitterly resentful. Having had no physical contact for years, she did not feel she could possibly care for him if he needed personal attention. He felt the same way, but had no one else to care for him, and at his age did not want to try to find institutional care to last until he died.

The arguments were not helped, because everyone who became involved took sides and, usually unasked, offered their own solutions. Margaret left and then returned and then left again. The final solution was not perfect; they divided the house in terms of living space, and she agreed to do the house duties and the cooking. She stayed at work to help pay for the extra care he might need as time passed. In return, he ensured that the house, which might have been divided, passed solely to her. They never became close. She did the absolute bare minimum for him, and they rarely spoke. Friends tried to help and again took sides. The situation was only resolved after some months by his rapid deterioration and sudden death.

Margaret openly admitted that she had been close to giving up such an intolerable situation, but felt she had no choice. She sold up and moved far away, and was eventually able to feel that there was no one person to blame, and that she had coped as well as she could. She had given him the care that he needed, but none of the affection. Perhaps it was easier for her since they had no real friends in common, and no children.

In a similar situation Glenda, aged sixty-one, left her husband Bill, and had no further contact, as she felt the bad relationship they had was a joint responsibility, and was not only her fault. It was hard on him as he was frightened, and wanted her to be there for him. For her it was just too late. She could not face a long drawn-out illness at her age, and wanted to build her new life as soon as possible. Their one daughter managed to stay friends with both Glenda and Bill and gave as much help as she could.

Patsy was only thirty when Gavin developed multiple sclerosis and was very quickly chair-bound, and helpless. At thirty-seven he was admitted to a long-term residential unit for full care. Patsy had care of the two children, both under ten. She went back to teaching, and seemed to be able to cope well. However, she had a separate life, a secret life away from the family, for a night a week, clubbing and generally having 'fun'.

She visited Gavin two or three times a week, brought the children at least once, always looked pretty and was well dressed. He loved seeing them, and was very proud of his family. Many people felt very critical of Patsy, when she began to be seen around on her night off by other visitors and some of the staff, and the gossip started. But she made no apology. She felt she did all she could to keep him happy, and it was nobody's business but her own.

Coming to Terms With Feelings of Guilt and Responsibility

However, it is hard not to feel responsible for a partner, close friend or relative when they are ill, and however good the level of care may be, carers find it hard to take time out and detach themselves from the situation. Both men and women can be tormented with guilt, but men are often more likely to be able to pay for care, simply because they have the financial means. This means that they are more able to detach physically from the everyday grind.

Leaving the situation for whatever reason often leaves the carer with feelings of guilt, which are very hard to forget, and can carry on for many years. So any decision to leave has to be taken with great thought and care. Decisions to stay must consider the needs of the carer for space, and time off, and provide defined boundaries.

Changes in a Mental State Such as Alzheimer's Disease

When there are psychological changes, either accompanying the illness or developing separately, as with Alzheimer's disease, or confusion, or dementia, which can occur with illnesses like AIDS, the carer has added problems, and sometimes it is impossible to continue with the care at home. People with mental health problems can become increasingly demanding and often uncooperative, and the main carer feels more and more trapped. Because of the shortage of beds for these patients, many of them stay at home for longer than the carer feels able to manage. The patient can often cover up their symptoms to outsiders for short periods at a time, making the level of dementia less apparent, even to professionals. Then the carer will need special support from those people around them, when they finally cannot manage, and request that the patient be admitted to a home, or hospital.

It is always better to investigate the illness to get as firm a diagnosis as possible, rather than accept the condition without investigation. A state of confusion or dementia is not necessarily Alzheimer's disease, though for the carer the difference may be seen as entirely unimportant. But symptoms can be very different indeed, and understanding them can help. Get a name for the disease because then there may be specialist advice to help, or some palliative treatment, and at the very least there will be some understanding of the prognosis and more chance to plan ahead.

Mike was the main carer for his wife Louise, who had early Alzheimer's disease, when he himself developed cancer, and he began to realise that he was not going to be able to care for her as he had planned. Unable to refuse her pleas not to leave her, he struggled on, refusing all offers of treatment and of help. Louise hated all visitors, and was especially suspicious of the hospice nurse, whom she suspected (quite rightly) of trying to take Mike away. Finally he collapsed; Louise was taken into a psychiatric ward as an emergency, and Mike to the hospice where he died almost immediately, still frantically worrying about his wife. The hospice team promised to follow her up afterwards and see if they could do anything for her.

It took a month for Louise to settle down in a nursing home, during which time she was very distressed and cried a lot of the time. However, when the hospice nurse visited she was surprised when Louise half-recognised her as a vaguely familiar face. When the nurse mentioned Mike, Louise said, 'He died years and years ago – this is my husband now,' waving her hand at a man sitting near her.

The nursing staff said that when he was admitted, she had bonded on sight with the other patient, and now thought she was married to him. As long as he was within reach she was amenable and friendly, even to his wife, when his family visited. It seemed sad that Mike was not able to see her settled, in time for him to have had some symptom control, and peace of mind, before he died.

Alzheimer's disease can present with many different symptoms. The only absolute is that it will continue to progress. It becomes very hard for the carer to believe that this is the same person they once knew, and harder still to believe that the patient is not deliberately being difficult, but that they truly cannot help themselves. The patient can be so cunning and manipulative that it seems impossible to believe that they are really unable to help their condition. No one who has not experienced close contact with a person with Alzheimer's can judge the difficulties, and the carer needs tremendous support in whatever solution they find for themselves.

As we have seen, Alzheimer's disease is not the only cause of mental changes. Some drugs can cause confusion or psychosis however carefully the team consider the medication. Some neurological diseases can result in psychological change and this is something that, on diagnosis, causes great fear and apprehension. This is another reason to ask and record questions and answers from the specialist.

The Alzheimer's Disease Society can offer support and advice and some insight into coping strategies for the carer, whatever the cause of the condition. In general they have a better understanding of this sad condition than many healthcare workers do.

There is a compassionate and honest book about the experiences of caring for a relative with MID or Multi-Infarct Dementia, which is sometimes confused with Alzheimer's disease, entitled *Remind Me Who I Am Again* by Linda Grant (ISBN 1-86207-171-3)

Margaret Forster has also written a moving and often funny book called *Have The Men Had Enough?* which gives insight into the difficulties of caring for someone who is confused or demented. A current carer may not find it so amusing but it is sympathetic and thoughtful. The book reference is ISBN 0-140-12769-0 published by Penguin books.

Trying to Understand When Faced With a Confused Relative

Confusion is not an illness, it is only a symptom. It is not the same as dementia, though demented patients can also become confused. A high proportion of patients with terminal illness experience some slight confused or muddled state. Sudden acute confusion or delirium can be due to drugs, infection and high temperature, severe pain, constipation, breathing difficulties and some heart problems. Generally if someone suddenly becomes unexpectedly confused, it is worth asking the professionals about common causes like new medication, or constipation. People who become constipated or dehydrated can appear very muddled and confused. People with brain tumours and AIDS do develop symptoms of confusion at times. Keeping an accurate chart over the preceding days is useful, and can sometimes pinpoint the start of the problem.

If someone becomes confused it is often tempting to collude with them, but sometimes this only encourages the confusion. It is generally better for the patient to be gently reminded of the true situation without scaring them, or making them distressed or aggressive. Sometimes explaining the confusion in simple terms and truthfully can help. For example:

'No, so-and-so is not here – he is at school/work...', or perhaps even 'He died a long time ago – do you remember?'

Obviously if someone asks the same question repeatedly

and gets terribly upset at the news each time, another answer has to be considered, but in general it is better to try and tell the truth instead of joining in with the lie.

'Remember, we gave you some new pills, and we thought they might make you a bit muddled. It will soon get easier for you.'

'This is not a hotel but you are in your own bed – see, there is the mirror etc.'

It is hard for the carer to find they are no longer recognised, and have to remind the patient who they are, and even what is their relationship. However, the patient will also be anxious and frightened by the confusion, and may be glad to be reminded that they are with someone who loves them and knows them.

Confusion should be investigated as soon as possible, as it is frightening and disturbing for everyone concerned. It is usually possible to make the situation better, if not completely cured.

If the local palliative care team are not actively involved in the care, the GP can always ask them for advice and suggestions, if he or she has trouble finding an answer to a problem, and the family do not want any hospice involvement.

Again, see the Appendix for other information.

Chapter Fourteen

Acknowledging Anger

Anger is a natural response to frustration and helplessness. A carer can be angry in response to the illness itself, or in response to the way it is being dealt with by the person with the illness, or by the family, or by the professionals. A person who is ill has many reasons to feel angry – because of their lost opportunities, and their lost dreams and hopes for the future. Whatever the cause it is healthier to explode regularly than to keep a tight rein on painful emotions. Acknowledging anger releases the emotion, and frees more energy to deal with daily life. Trying to remain a saint throughout illness is impossible for carer and patient alike.

People face situations differently, and there cannot be one answer to any situation. Some sick people will never come to terms with so much change, or find any comfort in doing anything that has never been of interest to them before. This can mean that the carer becomes the focal point of their existence, and a lifeline to them for the duration of the disease or illness. This can put a great strain on the carer, and on the relationship, and can leave the carer completely depleted. Trying to talk openly from the start of this experience can help to reduce rage building up because there is no outlet for the emotion.

Examples of Dealing With Anger

Some people will work out an individual way to alleviate the stress of all the negative emotions. Sometimes physical work is a release. Penny dug the garden in a passion, which her husband observed and remarked on when she finally came indoors. It made them both laugh initially, and then they wept in shared frustration. They both felt better and it became a family joke. 'Don't annoy her or she'll attack the garden again.'

Some people direct all their anger at the medical team who made the diagnosis, and are continuing the care or the treatment. Of course there may be good reason to feel angry, and that needs to be addressed. It is far more difficult to be angry with God, life, the illness or even the person who is ill, and so, sometimes, a family will take exception to one or other of the specialists, and they will join forces to direct all their anger at that person. A carer will often focus on something else to rage about: the neighbours, the government, family members, anything to be able to release some of the tension. Many professionals are aware of the reason for this displaced anger, and help each other to deal with their response, but many are very shocked by the level of rage they experience.

Strong Emotions Are Tiring

Anger and anxiety use up a lot of energy. Tiredness is the natural state when someone is fixed in a very stressful and angry situation. The carer cannot expend their mixed emotions on the patient, who already feels only too aware that they are the cause of all the trouble. Understanding this does not make it easier to manage, but sometimes if the carer is encouraged to talk about the stress, and the injustice in their own circumstances, some of the pent-up emotions are released.

Mark (from Chapter Five) was lucky to have an understanding teacher with whom he was able to play a mean game of squash when he felt frustrated. Another young man, Neil, started playing football and became a keen and noisy supporter of Arsenal, and his interest was a source of pleasure to him for many years after his parent had died.

Lily, in her late forties, found that when her husband was ill he could not rest unless she was within earshot and sight of him, twenty-four hours a day. He had always been possessive and quite jealous, and she had liked that aspect of their relationship, but it became a great strain when she felt under a microscope all the time. If she worked in the garden she had to leave the window open and stay where he could see her, or he banged on the window with his stick. No visitors were welcome. Her anger and frustration were building up, but when her friends urged her to sort him out she explained, 'This cannot go on for very long, and I know that no one will ever love me as absolutely and totally as he does. It may drive me mad now but when it is all over I know I will miss being the centre of someone's life even if I also enjoy the freedom.'

She chose to deal with him in that way and it worked for them for the short time she nursed him.

Len, caring for Alice who had Alzheimer's disease as well as breast cancer, was feeling totally cramped by the needs of his wife. Alice, who had always been quite demanding, could not be left at any time without pitiful bouts of weeping. The strain was exacerbated by her mental condition, which deteriorated faster than the cancer. He risked a huge argument, and very little sympathy from the rest of his family, when he demanded some free time and was not prepared to negotiate.

The result was an agreement that he should have one free afternoon each week – not a lot of time off for someone giving such continuous care and support. However, having made a stand he felt very much more confident, and after a few weeks of silent condemnation the imbalance in their relationship lessened, and his family seemed to give more thought to his needs. The family, now more involved with caring for their mother, began to realise how hard it was for Len, and were consequently more responsive to his needs.

Len tried to understand her mental condition. As we have seen, Alzheimer's disease often leaves only a glimpse of the real person there for the carer, and Len found it very hard to cope with this change. He did feel less resentful and less pressurised, as he recognised the fear behind her demands. He was genuine in his desire to care for her, but he needed to have a break regularly.

Many charities and carers associations offer a small break, for coffee and a chat at centres, where the carers can explode safely. It is good to be able to complain about not being appreciated, to threaten to leave, to wish it was all over and done with, and to moan about one's nearest and dearest, knowing that when you have finished speaking, nothing has been recorded and no one has been hurt. Much of the anger results from helplessness and the feelings of injustice at the illness.

Talking to the Right People

Unfortunately family members are not always the best people to have a moan to or at. They are too close to the situation to forget what has been said. Someone from outside, and therefore distanced from the problem, can listen and forget and not feel tempted to repeat. Few people really mean all they say when they are angry.

Graham's wife, Julia, was very conscious that her life was also passing her by. She had great plans for picking up her career, and embarking on further training, once the children were in full-time school. She often felt that she could not see an end to her problems. Even when he died she would find it hard to manage the children on her own, with less money, and no helping hand from Graham.

She talked freely to her sister, but her sister found it hard to listen without making judgements. She would remind Julia that Graham was going to die, and that he would have done the same for her had she been ill. She could not simply allow Julia the space to grumble and to feel a little sorry for herself, without judging her. Julia's brother-in-law, with whom she had never really bonded, was the one person who could just listen. He never made her feel guilty, and never reminded her later on that she had nursed such resentment. He was also able to refrain from encouraging her anger, by losing his temper as well. He was the perfect support for her.

It is normal to feel angry. It is normal for the anger to continue to appear throughout the illness and on into bereavement. It is not something to feel guilty about. Sharing the anger with the patient or with friends or family is often helpful and comforting.

The Emphasis on Accepting Any Help Available

As said previously, planning regular breaks or respite care for the family can prevent some of the anger and frustration from taking over. It gives a different environment for a short time, allows a change of company and shows a measure of appreciation for the carer. It also means there is something to look forward to, which breaks the monotony.

Unfortunately this is not often an option immediately on offer when someone is first diagnosed. Nor is it discussed in any detail soon after diagnosis. If it is offered by far-thinking social services, the family often reject the whole idea, caught up as they are in the emotional stress of the moment. In the immediate days after the diagnosis a potential carer will often feel they must be all things to all people, and fuelled with a desperate need to do *something*, they are not ready to consider a time when they may feel they cannot manage any longer. Often the potential patient is already worried about the effect that long-term caring will have on the spouse or partner, and so is very ready to look at options that can relieve the situation.

This is why in an ideal situation the opportunity of respite care should be talked through early on in the disease, and the couple encouraged to adopt that idea with their day-to-day plans. This means the idea becomes familiar at a time when the sick person is more fully aware of the needs of other people, and less frightened of leaving the security of the home and familiar carers. This is where hospice care can be very helpful, either as an inpatient for a short spell, or for support at home. Find out what is available from your local unit. People with AIDS have, over the years, evolved a 'buddy' system whereby a volunteer called a buddy will undertake to support and befriend someone, throughout their illness. This buddying can be immensely rewarding for all the people concerned, as well as very sad at times.

Helen and Jim were in their late forties when he was diagnosed with cancer of the stomach. He was quite ill by the time he was diagnosed, having ignored his symptoms for as long as possible, because he had been reluctant to stop working. He had been a car mechanic all his life and still loved his job.

They asked to be in contact with their local hospice very early after his diagnosis. He asked if he could spend a day every two weeks in the day care unit where he soon began to know the medical and nursing staff well and he felt at home. He had no further hospital appointments, unless he requested them, so the hospice took over his care totally. Part of the point of day care was to give Helen a rest, and as the months went by he started to have the occasional short spell in the unit and was quite happy with that service. His proudest day came when he was able to talk the hospice odd job man through a car problem, and solve it from his wheelchair.

Jim's cancer developed more slowly than was expected, and so he was able to talk at length to the staff there, and he became very calm, and no longer so frightened about his diagnosis and general condition.

Hospice Care as an Inpatient

The disadvantage of a long stay in the hospice is that regular visitors see quite a few people die over the weeks, and this can be quite depressing. This is an aspect that has to be taken into consideration when planning combined inpatient and outpatient care. The advantage is that a person feels confident about staying there because they know how it works, and who will be caring for them, and the care offered is not impersonal, as are hospital admissions. Jim and Helen were treated as a unit and when she started to become very tired he was glad to accept the offer of a week respite care, while she had a holiday, and she felt happy to leave him there, knowing he was receiving the best of care. He died at home however, in his own bedroom, as he always wanted.

Hospice is not the only option. There are several charities, as well as religious organisations, that offer help and respite care, and some of these are listed below. The main thing is to consider the idea and plan on using the option *before* the carer becomes exhausted and it becomes an emergency situation.

Holidays

There are also many people who long for a holiday, and would love to have one together if there were help available.

Sometimes a family can team up, and with several people helping they can have a relaxing and very happy holiday in resorts that cater for disabled people. This can be hard for a sick person to cope with, as it is easy to feel resentful when it is impossible to escape the knowledge that everyone concerned now knows the extent of their disability. Paul, with a severe and rapid motor neurone disease, went on holiday with a group of ten of his extended family, and his wife and three children. He spent the first week raging at his helplessness, but then gave up, and was able to accept all help, bar that of his mother. He simply could not cope with her pushing his wheelchair, and helping to feed him. It felt too much like being a baby again.

Strangely, his four-year-old son elected to help to feed him, and this was quite acceptable to Paul, and continued throughout his illness, giving the little boy a sense of importance, as well as giving Paul and the family a lot of amusement. The child, who had been quite fussy about his food, developed a healthy appetite, and mealtimes became an important part of the day and were associated with laughter and fun. Paul came close to choking when he was told 'Open wide, Daddy.'

Sometimes a whole family can get together to help with travel arrangements. This can be a great support to the family and also good fun and a source of happy memories later on.

Talking With Children

Children of all ages are often very angry, especially when they are not included and informed and they ask questions that are left unanswered or inadequately answered. Any emotional tensions affect even very small children. Allowing them the time to voice their insecurities and frustrations can lessen the problems at a later date. This does not mean a constant pressure to talk, but offering an appreciation of how they feel – a comment such as 'It must be very hard for you to see all this pain going on and still have to behave as if everything is OK when you are at school,' or 'How are your friends acting – are you able to talk to them, or do you feel they don't really understand or want to talk about it?' or 'How are you managing to sleep with such a lot on your mind?' or 'Is there anything you don't understand or is there anything that we/I can do to make it a bit easier or clearer for you?'

It isn't the words that matter but giving a child or young person the understanding that it is not unusual to feel pretty low and helpless and they do not have to be super brave all the time. Nor do they have to feel guilty for wishing it were not happening/wishing it would soon be all over/wishing they could disappear and avoid the whole thing. These are normal emotions.

Chapter Fifteen

Dealing With Depression and Isolation

Depression is not the same as sadness. It is normal to feel sad in the midst of tragedy. Sadness comes and goes, and can be talked through, wept through and subsides. Depression can be a lot harder to understand and help.

This chapter is not meant to be a clinical explanation of depression. There are complex factors leading to depression.

Most people accept that a degree of depression is common with the shock of receiving, and adjusting to, a diagnosis of terminal illness. Sometimes it is a temporary state that passes quickly, with or without treatment, but can return. People can become depressed when they are seemingly quite well, and living much longer than at first expected. It is not always possible to differentiate between natural sadness and depression. *It could be said that sadness is overwhelming emotion, but depression is almost total lack of emotion.* The immediate cause of either state is often the lack of any definite future. Uncertainty is very hard to live with.

Surprisingly it is not uncommon for people who have always experienced depression without apparent cause, to cope heroically when they are faced with something like terminal illness, if it is happening to them and not to someone close to them.

Depression and Anti-depressants

Sometimes someone's depression can never be resolved. Anti-depressants can be useful, but any medication has side effects, and these may make it hard for the sick person to persevere with new medication. And anti-depressants have to be taken on a regular basis, not when, and if, someone remembers. Some take fourteen days or longer to start to have an effect. Some side effects are minimal, and can easily be ignored. More severe effects like constipation should be anticipated, and, again, a good GP will advise, and taking a mild laxative will avoid complications. Once again the best way to make a decision is to talk to your specialist if they prescribe anti-depressants, and come to a joint decision.

It is always a good idea to ask the pharmacist to comment when starting new medication, as they almost always have a very wide knowledge of the effects of medication. This is not to undermine the role of the GP but very often doctors do not check the compatibility of the drugs in a mixture of medication. This can happen when there are several doctors prescribing for one person, like a GP and an oncologist/neurologist or consultant. As we saw in Chapters Eight and Ten, a very useful tip is to make up a drug chart, which can be shown to the pharmacist as well as to other professionals, and will enable them to see at a glance what is being taken.

This also enables the family to remember the reason for giving the medication, and again this can be very helpful if there are several people involved in the care. It is very easy to overdose or under-dose when people are not used to taking medication, and are trying to adjust to a new routine.

Sometimes depression responds to counselling, but the patient must be ready to consider this route. Counselling is not like a treatment, but rather a two-way process, requiring full co-operation from the patient. It cannot be inflicted on someone, especially if they are exhausted and unwilling.

Perhaps the most difficult situation to come to terms with is when, after a long spell of hospitals and diagnosis, and then inactivity, it becomes apparent that the original diagnosis is wrong, or that there will not be a definite diagnosis at all. Or perhaps the original diagnosis is overshadowed by complications that may or may not be associated with the illness.

As we have seen, life changes so much and very suddenly. There are many new people like the professional team visiting; there are complete changes in routine; and hopefully increased help in the house, as well as extra equipment. All of this adds up to an invasion of privacy, and a feeling of loss of control.

With so little control over one's life, it is easier to understand why someone should give up the effort to make any sense of it. Once depression sets in it is almost impossible to arouse any interest in the events of day-to-day living. Open discussion with the GP or specialist is essential, as the person in the centre of the problem may have no idea that they are depressed.

The Wrong Diagnosis

As said previously, there are sometimes cases of misdiagnosis among some neurological diseases. If little is known about a disease the rate of progression of the disease may be uncertain, and the family can feel very bewildered. Yet having become used to the diagnosis, and made all the necessary plans and adjustments, to find that everything seems to have changed can be as upsetting as the initial diagnosis. As we have seen, the original label becomes the patient's identification and they have often become an expert in their disease.

Greg was aged thirty-nine when he became ill, had become very used to his original diagnosis of multiple sclerosis, and was initially told that he had a short prognosis. He had deteriorated fast in the first year after he was diagnosed but very little in the following six years. He became increasingly depressed and difficult to live with. Meg had given up her job at the beginning to care for him as he deteriorated, and they had both become experts in their field, doing voluntary work for the associated charity and attending all support-group activities.

After seven years they had seen many newfound friends die, many changes in the provision of care, and new faces coming and going in the carers they were offered. In some ways he no longer fitted into the original diagnosis, and yet he was reluctant to undergo more tests to see if there had been a mistake.

When he finally saw a different consultant, he was told that no one could be certain of his condition, but that he could consider himself fortunate to have outlived so many others. Greg did not feel fortunate at all. He felt useless and, in a way fraudulent, for not having died like the other people he had met. His role within the charity support group became less clear, as he felt he did not meet the criteria anymore. Meg felt that her life was on hold, holidays put aside, career cut off. Friends had developed other interests, and visitors were often left frustrated by his depression and lack of response and gave up their visits. This is a common reaction, as depressed people do not make good company.

Living a Day at a Time

For people who have no definite diagnosis or a very rare and little-known disease, the psychological needs may be different, and the response of friends and family may vary. It is very hard to accept a diagnosis when no one knows anything about it at the best of times, and many people with a rare disease become increasingly frustrated at having to explain their problems in detail to every caller. It is even more difficult when there is nothing to explain, and no way of anticipating the next step, or when there is an underlying illness that may not be identified for some time, and is completely unexpected.

Gloria and Frank, both in their mid-sixties and young for their age, accepted his diagnosis of bowel cancer, and were adjusting well to the changed circumstances. However, she found his frequent memory lapses, and odd bouts of inexplicable behaviour, very much more difficult to deal with. He could be aggressive and resist all suggestions, and then gracefully capitulate and appear to have no memory of his tantrum. The specialist was not really interested in something other than his cancer, and strangers were not so aware of the changes in personality that were so obvious to Gloria. When he had a final assessment, the diagnosis of Alzheimer's disease meant she eventually had him placed in a unit where he could be safe and given proper care.

She was quite unable to associate this new Frank with the tranquil and beloved partner of more than forty years, and she felt very guilty at her inability to manage him at home, where in his rational moments he wanted to be. She made good use of the support available, but was never able to accept fully what she felt was the way she had let him down. She was deeply depressed for many weeks. Medication helped her to accept that some situations are not fully resolvable, and that the only sensible decision was the one she had taken.

She and Frank were fortunate indeed that they were able to get a place for him. As we have already said, it is very difficult to manage any dementia at home, without a great deal of help. When it is coupled with an illness that requires co-operation from the patient, it becomes almost impossible.

This is a problem that is being recognised by the authorities, and should mean more help in the future. For the present the carer will need an advocate to push for more help and respite care at very regular intervals. This is often fiercely opposed by the patient, which adds to the guilt.

Marc and David, who were in a long-term relationship and had lived together for many years, coped well when David had surgery for his early diagnosis of lung cancer. However, it became obvious that this was not his only problem, as it took so long for him to recover from surgery. When they discovered he also had a form of neurological disease they were absolutely shocked and both found it very hard to see any hope at all in the future.

When Talking Helps

For a small group of people, disability can bring back memories that have been buried deep for very good reasons, and that can be very destructive. Albert, in his eighties, had been a prisoner of war for four years when he was young, and had never been able to talk about his experiences. When his weakness and disability became severe, he began to experience distressing recall of some of the horrors of those years. He dreamed he was being beaten and ill treated, and awoke very frightened and disorientated. These flashbacks led to deep depression, and a feeling of guilt that he had lived so much longer than his comrades. This is not an uncommon reaction among older people who did not have the benefit of the understanding or counselling that nowadays is offered routinely, following any experience in a crisis or major disaster.

Albert's GP was very understanding, and was able to prescribe medication and mild sedatives to help him relax enough to go to sleep. The surgery had a counsellor attached to the practice, who was able to talk to him for some time over a few weeks, until the memories were laid to rest as far as possible. He was never completely free of them, and often dreaded going to sleep. Albert was very fortunate in the help that was available. Sometimes the war veterans' associations or the Royal British Legion can be very helpful if the patient can identify the cause of the nightmares.

Milly, also in her eighties, had a very tragic childhood. Ill treated, neglected and hungry, she had not known any affection or care until she met and married Sid, when she was sixteen years old. She thought she had buried her past in her happy and protected marriage, but her illness brought the sadness and fear and helplessness flooding back. She found that talking to her grandchild, also aged sixteen, was a great comfort to her, and she was able to unburden herself in a way she had never been able to previously. The granddaughter was absolutely fascinated and wrote down all she was told, which made a remarkable record for all the family, many of whom were scattered widely, and were not all aware of the sad history of their grandmother

Most people, whatever their history, find that talking about it can help to lay the ghosts. However, many cannot bring themselves to do so, and it is not productive to probe and force confidences, which must be given freely. This is where support groups can help sometimes, when there is camaraderie borne out of past experiences, which may never be fully understood by those who have not had similar experiences.

For people who feel they have wasted lives and wasted opportunities, there is the realisation that there will not be time to make amends. Sometimes, just talking this through helps and can also identify values that have been overlooked and unrecognised.

Sometimes complementary therapy can offer solutions. Aromatherapy or homeopathy can have quite powerful effects, and some natural remedies have been found to be therapeutic for depression, without the side effects associated with anti-depressants. Also, the personal attention implicit in performing these therapies, particularly when physical contact is involved, can help to make a depressed person feel valued and appreciated.

Many doctors will have a negative response to complementary therapies, but some people find great relief in such practices, which can help with the emotional pain. Many of these complementary therapies have been used effectively for many years without a certificate approving them. It seems a shame to ignore or reject such practices, if there is a possibility of using them to benefit someone.

Massage is a therapeutic tool that can also relieve stress and anxiety, and it is well worth considering such options, as well as traditional medical solutions.

Some people find a way to do something that really makes them feel as if they have achieved something of importance during their life. James became evangelistic about giving up smoking and felt huge achievement if he convinced someone to stop the habit.

When there is guilt over a past regret, writing a letter or letters makes someone feel they have tidied up the loose ends to an extent, and they can do no more. There can be great peace of mind when the loose ends are tied, and it is well worth the effort.

Sometimes it has to be accepted that there is not going to be a solution for some people who become depressed. The only way to cope is to take the situation day by day. Living with someone who is depressed is hard indeed, and the entire family unit needs support and understanding, and regular time out of the situation, if that is at all possible.

Chapter Sixteen

The Question of Euthanasia and Suicide

In our western culture, whenever death is discussed in any depth, the subject of euthanasia is mentioned. In parts of Europe in recent years, some doctors have been advocating patient choice for people who believe it is their right to die when they wish. The churches are usually opposed to the idea, as are many other people who feel that this acceptance may lead to society pressurising people to request death, rather than become a burden to society and their family. It is not legal in this country to assist in the death of a person, however ill they may be and however they request the help. It is feared that legalising euthanasia will lead to undue pressure being applied on weak and helpless people to ask for help to die.

There is quite a strong lobby advocating euthanasia in this country and there are several websites supporting and advising people who are looking for a choice. It may be that attitudes will change in the future, but at the time of writing this book, it is not an option in the United Kingdom.

Professionals do not give large doses of medication like morphine in order to kill someone, but of course all medication has some side effects, and sometimes death is so close that the medication may appear to precipitate death. As stated in Chapter Seventeen there is always someone who will give the last injection, the last wash, the last drink, or the last kiss. With minimal medication there will always be those last actions. No medication is intended to cause death. But to omit the injection or the pill may cause distress, perhaps pain, perhaps acute agitation, and that is therefore not an option, since the hope is to ensure a peaceful and gentle death.

For many carers, whether family, friends or professionals the last few weeks of a life can be immensely rewarding, and can remove all fear of death from those left behind.

There cannot be an answer to satisfy everyone, but often people who work with the dying are asked the question 'Will you give me something to end all this?' Most of those who ask are frightened, in pain or some discomfort, and most believe things can only get worse. Some think they are doing the family a kindness by relieving them of a burden. Many are terrified that things will get worse and they will not be able to bear whatever is to come.

Carers are also asked to help end a life, which the patient feels has become unbearable. All too often the carer cannot face the question and brushes it aside unanswered, only to relive it over again, for years afterwards, wondering if there should have been an answer.

Giving an Honest Answer

If the question can be acknowledged and answered, there is some feeling of completion in the situation.

The way a person makes the request indicates the degree of despair in which they find themselves. To ask to be 'done away with' or 'put down' shows the feelings of worthlessness and anger, only just below the surface. This is a hard request for anyone, and harder still when it comes from someone very much loved and needed.

Sometimes it is said that a dog would be put down in such a situation. However, most people would not equate the life of their parent or loved one, with the life of a dog.

As we have said, usually when someone asks to die it is because they want relief from all that they are suffering, mentally and physically. So if relief can be given, together with the recognition that they are going to die in time anyway, and that this situation is not going to drag on forever, many people will no longer wish to be killed, but will accept that death will come in the allotted time. For most people the feeling that this experience is endless is the worst part of the illness.

There is also the fear that things might get even worse with more pain and unpleasant symptoms, perhaps some that cannot be controlled. People often believe there is a limit to the medication that can be given. In fact symptom relief is a highly expert field and it is rare that the situation cannot be improved. Medical teams are more than willing to share and exchange solutions, to help people in need.

Knowing that there is a limit to life, that it is possible to keep a person comfortable and relatively pain-free, can be very reassuring. Many people believe that everyone has some influence in the timing of their own death. This is discussed further in Chapter Seventeen, Dying at Home.

It is likely that more people kill themselves than we realise. People known to be in the last stages of a terminal illness are not subject to a post mortem if they die suddenly, and have been seen recently by the doctor, and they often have the medication at hand to hurry things along. When AIDS first became known, and it was felt that there was little anyone could do to make the patients more comfortable, many people believed that a large number of people with the disease committed suicide. Fortunately this may not happen so frequently now the disease is better understood and far more manageable.

Fear of Having Life Prolonged Can Cause Anxiety

Many people find that by talking to their doctor, and getting reassurance that he will not attempt to prolong the life of the sick person, is all the reassurance they need. Again it is a question of honest open discussion. It is quite legal for the medical team to agree with the family that there will be no medication given with the intention of prolonging their life. For example, sometimes prescribing an antibiotic for a chest infection for someone who is near to death does not help their quality of life and may extend life for a very short and miserable time. However in a slightly different case it may ease discomfort and add to their quality. So ask questions and talk to the doctor and get their opinion.

Every suicide involves other people. Someone has to contribute in some way, usually unknowingly or unexpectedly, to the death, and someone has the shock of finding the body afterwards.

Suicide is hard for families and friends to accept. Even distant friends feel guilty and wish they had done something. Often family, especially the younger members, feel guilty, since they are sure they could have prevented it had they been more aware.

It is very difficult indeed to commit suicide, and leave everyone feeling much happier. The guilt remains. Even professionals will remember for years the person who killed themselves while in their care.

So if suicide is mentioned it seems healthier to discuss it within the family, and at least get a consensus of opinion before making further plans. There can never be a perfect way of dealing with the wish to die.

Here are some examples of how other people managed –

and how the families felt afterwards. None of these examples is meant as a criticism, but merely to show the different ways in which people have dealt with the wish to die.

Rose was a secondary school teacher of maths and sciences, and was fifty-two when she became ill with a rapidly developing ovarian cancer. She had always been very correct, and her family of husband Nicholas and two adult daughters seemed close, but were not at all demonstrative. Nicholas had always been a workaholic, burying himself in his business. Neither Rose nor Nicholas appeared to encourage neighbours to pop in. Professional carers who briefly met the couple were all aware of the formal atmosphere in the house. The daughters lived nearby but neither had married. Rose seemed to keep them all at an emotional distance.

Without giving any apparent warning, she took an overdose of sleeping tablets.

She was found by her cleaning lady, who called the emergency services – she was taken to hospital and recovered. She was sent home with the promise of a counsellor within a few weeks. Rose was very depressed. She was reluctant to eat, she spoke little, grew unkempt and careless about her looks, and the rift in the family widened. The family seemed to guard her, making sure she was never left alone. All her medication was hidden. She became more frustrated daily as she grew weaker. She refused to discuss her feelings with anyone, only repeating over again that she wanted to die.

She then planned to drown herself but was caught outside and taken home again. After that she was locked in. She died very quickly, quite unexpectedly, having never spoken freely to anyone about her fears. Her family felt completely desperate, and could not come to terms with their feeling of failure. Both daughters left the area soon after she died, and barely made contact with each other after that. Some time later the younger girl attempted suicide herself. The family home was sold soon after her death and her husband moved away to a new house.

Try to Find Someone to Listen

Jeanette was also in her early fifties when she was diagnosed with an incurable cancer of the bowel. She had three daughters and a very quiet and thoughtful husband. In the early days after the diagnosis she felt ill and very tired all the time, but was not in any pain. She also felt depressed and frightened of the future.

She raised the question of euthanasia with the district nurse, who felt unable to discuss it with her, and could not offer any advice, other than she should not do it. She confided to some of her friends that she had no wish to keep on living, but they all sidetracked the issue, and she was not able to discuss it openly with anyone.

She finally managed to talk to the ward sister on one of her short hospital visits. This person said she should talk about her feelings with her family – having had a suicide in her own family, she had first-hand experience of the effect on those left behind.

Very reluctantly, but feeling increasingly desperate, Pat tried to talk to her eldest daughter when she visited that very afternoon. Lauren was twenty-three (Paula was twenty, and Ella was seventeen and still at school). Jeanette was surprised that Lauren was so upset by the conversation. She agreed that the ward was not the best place for such a discussion, and deferred the subject until she was in the privacy of her own home.

The first evening she was home the family gathered in the sitting room and had a conference. Jeanette was astonished at the strength of their distress, and even Edward her husband was vocal in expressing his feelings. She was also surprised to find that all the family had already made their own investigations into solutions and options for her situation. Lauren had visited the local hospice with her father, and they had talked at length to some of the staff there. Paula had phoned a cancer support group for information, which she had shared with Ella.

Jeanette was surprised and touched by their concern. She listened to all they said and agreed to visit the hospice, but did not want to read anything about her disease. She felt very defensive, and she clung to her belief that she alone had the right to make the decision to end her life.

Over the next few days the family talked a lot. They spent a lot of time together sharing information and feelings and supporting each other. As the days passed the heaviness in the house lightened, and their discussions were less emotional.

Jeanette finally agreed that she would do nothing for three months, during which time she would look for some options, and see how she felt generally. She would also allow her children to help to an extent with her care.

A month later she received a letter signed by the family stating that they loved her dearly, and wanted to be there for her as she had always been there for them; that they felt it an honour to look after her, but that if it became a chore and they felt that it was too much for any one of them they would be open with her, and ask for more help from Social Services. And if she decided she had had enough at some point, and wanted to die, they would support her in that wish and would not pressure her any further.

She became very calm as she grew weaker. Medication helped her symptoms a great deal. She had a short course of anti-depressants and felt a lot better. As her attitude changed, her family also relaxed, and they seemed to get a lot of pleasure from looking after her. She did not need anything like the level of care that she had anticipated, and so did not worry so much about being a burden.

She did not use the inpatient facilities of the hospice but accepted the regular visits from the palliative care team, without really allowing them to become emotionally very close to her. She understood that no one would force her to accept medication to prolong her life, and she felt very relieved by this. She no longer talked about suicide or being a burden.

She died peacefully at home fairly soon afterwards. All her family agreed that those months were very precious to them, and they felt accepting and grateful for that time. She had never mentioned suicide again.

Maria was a very deeply religious woman with seven children between the ages of eight and twenty-six. They were a happy and united family, though they had never been rich. Pete worked hard long hours as a bus driver. Maria managed the house and the budget and was the centre of the family.

When she was diagnosed with a brain tumour, she thought long and hard about her life and decided she would refuse all treatment, as she did not want to change her appearance at all. Neither did she want to be disabled and needing care for a long period. She felt that the disease should take its natural course, and treatment would delay the inevitable ending.

She stayed at home, happy and peaceful with regular visits from her priest. All her visitors were touched by the care her children gave her. They acted as a well-trained team, and supported each other. Pete had little to do in the way of organisation, but it was he who sat with her when he got home, and so the others were able to go their ways, and get some relief. His employers and all his workmates were very good to him, and helped to adjust his timetable so that he could work reasonable hours for a while.

Maria deteriorated and died very quickly, and until the very end she refused to take any treatment, other than the tablets to help relieve her headaches. Her family appeared to accept that she had done what she wanted, and her professional carers all felt that she had made the right decision for her particular circumstances.

Of course, it is much easier when an illness does not linger for a long time, and when the sick person does not change dramatically, and become a stranger, as we have seen with Alzheimer's disease.

Family circumstances also vary, and this has an effect. Not everyone has the support of a loving family, nor can everyone learn to talk in an open way about their innermost thoughts, if they have never done so before.

William was in his mid-seventies. He was a smart and sociable person, who liked a drink and a singsong with friends. He had spent a lifetime in the army, was used to travelling, but had settled well after he retired, and had formed a strong group of friends in the neighbourhood. His wife Gwen was a gentle person, who had always been his support and his best friend.

Cancer of the mouth robbed him of his speech very quickly. He felt it also robbed him of his close and affectionate physical relationship with Gwen. He no longer liked seeing friends. He hated being the quiet one and hated using the speaking aid he had been given because it seemed slow and lacked spontaneity. Although he could still communicate, in a fashion, he was not the same man, and he could see nothing in his future that could hold any attraction for him.

Unable to give full verbal expression to his feelings, he wrote a letter to Gwen and one to the stranger he planned to use to end his life. He then left home and stepped under a train.

No one could have blamed him, Gwen least of all, as she fully understood his state of mind when he did it. She only wished and continued to wish that she had been aware of his feelings and his plans, though she did not know what action she could possibly have taken to accept it or to prevent it. She might at the very least have had the opportunity to say goodbye. She felt especially sad when she thought that she would never know whether he might have regretted his action in those last few moments before he died. It seemed a brutal ending to a life that had been full and happy.

The After Effects on the Family

There cannot be any right or wrong about an individual action like suicide. But if everyone has the opportunity to talk it through with someone, then at least the person in the centre has the chance to see how people feel about them, and how important they are to someone. That has to be better than dying alone and perhaps feeling forgotten.

After Maria died Pete said that he would change nothing about the last year in spite of the sadness. The children resumed their lives easily, supporting each other when that was needed, and all talked about her with love and gratitude.

Edward also felt grateful and proud of the way his family had coped. He felt they could overcome anything in future. He said his only regret was that Jeanette would not be there for him when his time came.

Chapter Seventeen

Dying at Home

It is true that the vast majority of people express a desire to die at home. However, few actually achieve their wish. And when they do, the last few weeks of life are often plagued by anxiety about what will happen, whether they can cope with the experience, and what the family should do when death finally occurs.

Very few professionals visiting the home attempt to discuss the moment of death, for fear of causing distress, and sometimes because they too are not absolutely sure of what they would do in the same situation.

Families do not like to ask the question either, sometimes for fear of precipitating the death, or of appearing too eager to get it over. However, the silence can feel very intimidating as the family members worry individually, about what actually has to be done.

There are many useful and informative booklets about the legal requirements following a death at home. The legal requirements do not have to be dealt with urgently, and if death takes place during working hours, there are usually plenty of people around to direct and support the family. The dilemma comes with what to do in the practical sense, particularly since a large number of people die in the early hours of the morning, when the family may have no one present to support or help them. Giving some early thought to the situation can relieve a lot of anxiety, as well as making sure that whatever happens immediately after the death, the people present find comfort and support in their actions.

Each person dies just once. There are rarely 'practice runs', and each death is the completion of a very special life for someone. We pay great attention to giving birth, constantly reviewing the process and adapting responses to individual needs. Surely we should have the same attitude to dying? To have the opportunity to be at the side of someone we love when they leave us, is a great privilege, and it seems sad that the experience is often avoided through ignorance and fear.

Many people who have been present at the death of a loved one lose all fear of dying afterwards, and feel deep gratitude for having been able to be there.

The most important thing to know is that for most people, there is nothing to be afraid of in the process of dying, either for the person who is dying, or for the carer. Whether the disease has been rapid or slow, and however erratic the emotional response has been throughout the illness, the process of dying is usually calm and peaceful and accepting. People have compared it to the turn of the tide, or the change of seasons – barely perceptible, but immensely significant.

Of course there are always exceptions. Fear of pain, or other symptoms, and fear of an afterlife and a vengeful god, can all make the death more difficult. Expectations often affect the whole process, and sadly can result in some families describing terrible experiences of death. Some people do find it hard to die, but relatively few. Because symptoms are not understood or treated, the family become frightened, and they may misinterpret what is happening.

Common Questions

HOW MUCH CAN PEOPLE HEAR WHEN THEY ARE NEAR DEATH?

The last sense we lose is said to be hearing, and so it is important to remember when sitting with a loved one that some communication can often continue until the very last few moments.

Diane was forty-three and was a single mum for most of her daughter's childhood. There was never a lot of money around, but June was very much loved and Diane gave her all she could. They were very close but June had been a difficult teenager, and at nineteen was only just becoming easier to live with, when Diane was diagnosed with bowel and liver cancer. June was very supportive and cared for her mother devotedly, but Diane was so ill, so quickly, that there was not a lot of time to talk. The last three nights before she died they had a Marie Curie nurse with them all night, as June was looking very stressed and frightened.

The nurse sat by the bed, with June on the other side, and they each held a hand and watched silently as Diane lay there. Most of the time she neither moved nor spoke. Occasionally she became restless and muttered and moved around, and required small amounts of medication, or to have her bed changed, as she had become incontinent. June wept silently, intermittently, and said little.

When June did begin to talk, Diane made no response. June told the nurse she had been a difficult teenager, and how sad she felt now and how she wished she had the time over again to make it up to her mother. She grieved that she would never be able to tell her mother all the things she appreciated about her, and that all she was left with were memories of her own bad behaviour for the last four years or so.

The nurse told her this.

'Your mother was also sixteen once. She was probably just as bad as you were. She may have been even worse. We all argue with our parents, and we give them as hard a time as we can while we are finding our feet. Most of us are lucky because we grow older and have time to make up for the bad times, and can laugh about them later. Some of us are still laughing when our grandchildren are sixteen, and we watch it all start again with the daughters of our daughters.

'The worst thing your mother could know would be that you will carry this with you for the rest of your life. If she could speak she would tell you that she loves you, and that you have been a joy as well as a pain, and she would not have been without you. She wants you to be happy, she is proud of the way you have coped through her illness, she would hate you to have such regrets.'

At this point Diane suddenly gripped their hands till they hurt. And then she gave a broad smile. She did not open her eyes or say a word. Not long afterwards she died. It was as if she felt it had all been said. Neither June nor the nurse had any doubt at all that Diane knew what was being said.

Brenda, a fifty-year-old single woman, had a fearful time with abdominal surgery for her bowel cancer, followed by treatments that all seemed to go wrong in one way or another. She fought the progression of her illness with implacable rage, and as she became weaker her friends felt helpless in the face of her fear and frustration. Two days before her death she suddenly became calm and told the friend who was sitting with her:

'It's all OK now, you can let go my hand, I'm not frightened anymore. It will all be fine. Thank you for coming, please tell everyone not to worry about me.'

She slept quietly, talking only a little for the last few days but always calmly, and then died peacefully.

This is not an uncommon experience – as death becomes

inevitable, it is usual for the dying one to grow calm, and to appear to be at peace and unafraid.

Whatever the religious beliefs of the people concerned, for anyone able to be present at the end of a life is a moving and rewarding experience, and can be a source of great comfort to those who are left. The main thing to know is that there is no right or wrong behaviour, apart from what is defined in religious and cultural practices. The family is free to do whatever they feel comfortable doing.

In the rare instances when death appears to be more violent or distressing, the person dying seems to have no awareness of the distress, and indeed if they do speak they often associate the trauma with someone else.

WHAT ABOUT THE NOISES LIKE THE DEATH RATTLE?

May, aged eighty, was the eldest in a large family, and had bossed her siblings around all their lives, as she did her own four children. Her children adored her, but were still very obedient throughout her diagnosis of cancer, and supported her in her refusal to consider any treatment. She continued to control as much as possible until the last few days, when, surrounded by her family, she slept deeply most of the time, waking only for a few seconds now and then.

Towards the end of her life her breathing became so noisy that the family were very distressed and concerned for her. Suddenly she opened her eyes and said very clearly, 'Tell whoever that is making that row to get out of my room,' which caused unexpected and comforting amusement to the anxiously waiting family.

This noisy breathing usually causes more concern to the watchers by the bedside than to the person who is making the noise. It is commonly known as the 'death rattle' but it is simply fluids collecting along the entrance to the lungs. As the body slows down it can no longer clear the fluids away and so they rattle. It is possible to give drugs that will dry the excretions up, but may make the patient have a very dry mouth, and given the choice, some carers reject them.

Similarly the breathing also slows down, and the patient may miss a breath or two, and then start again. For the person watching this can be scary, as they keep thinking that death has finally come, and then with a big sigh, the breathing starts again. This is known as Cheyne-Stokes breathing and is perfectly natural as the body is slowly winding down, a little like a low-running battery. It does not appear to trouble the patient.

WHAT DOES IT MEAN WHEN SOMEONE KEEPS TUGGING AND PULLING AT THE BEDCLOTHES?

The other common condition to arise is called 'terminal restlessness'. The dying person's hands cannot keep still, they move constantly, tug at the bedclothes, perhaps they will mutter a lot, and appear very agitated. Holding their hands, stroking their head, talking softly, may have no effect and does not seem to calm them. This is not difficult to manage medically, and a palliative care team will plan for this, as it is a recognised and common experience. Betty, Alan's wife, mentioned earlier in this book, had a lovely explanation and interpretation for this condition, described further on in this chapter.

DO WE CALL THE EMERGENCY SERVICES?

It is important to realise that when an expected death happens there is no need to dial 999 and call out the emergency services. If they are called, the emergency services are bound to react, not knowing the person or their condition. When death is inevitable and anticipated, there is really nothing they can hope to achieve.

161

Sometimes, someone who has died can look really well, especially if they are young, and the immediate response when the emergency team arrive is to try and resuscitate. If there is any attempt at resuscitation, what might have been a gentle and quiet death can become noisy, aggressive and almost public. It is often very hard to accept that nothing more can be done to prolong a life. People still talk about a person 'fighting to live' whereas in fact many people might be said to be fighting to be allowed to die when their time is right.

DO WE HAVE ANY CONTROL OVER WHAT IS HAPPENING WHEN WE ARE DYING?

If this is something that has been talked about, so that the whole family are aware and supporting each other, then it is easier for the person who is dying to let go of life gracefully. Many people believe that giving the dying person permission to let go of life can ease the final moments, and give great comfort to the family. Often it can seem friends and family are holding onto someone who, if allowed, would be ready to let go. Sometimes a way of holding hands can give the impression of hanging on, and if the family are also saying 'Don't leave me,' which is an instinctive response at such a time, the powerful emotions in a room can cause tension.

Dave and Beryl had been married for thirty happy years and were very close. They were both diagnosed during the same week with cancer – a secondary cancer for Dave, but a new diagnosis for Beryl. The shock was very great for the family, but especially for their only daughter, who was in her late twenties. Over the following months Beryl did most of the caring, as Dave was already weak and ill. He was expected to live only a few weeks, but he remained alive, frail and ill and needing a lot of care, which he did not want anyone but Beryl to give.

Beryl became increasingly tired, and said to the visiting nurse that she was exhausted, and beginning to wish Dave would not hang on so long. She was frightened of what would happen when she was too unwell herself to care for him. She was becoming irritable and resentful that she also wanted some care and looking after. She longed for a good night's sleep, for a lie down in the afternoon, for someone to cook light meals for her. She felt as if she was unimportant, that her illness was taking a back seat. And she felt guilty for saying so.

The suggestion from the nurse was that Beryl tell Dave how she felt. That she tell him she loved him, that he had been a wonderful husband and father and that she would miss him, but that she was tired and weary and ill herself, and was now wondering how on earth they would manage. She had done all she could, was scared they would be physically separated if she became unable to continue, and that in effect he need not try so hard to stay with her, that he could let go. She thought about this and said that they had never talked like that to each other. It was suggested that she use her own words.

She went to his bed and took his hands and said, 'On your bike, Dave, love. You've been my best mate but I'm bloody shattered now, so get on with it.'

He gave her an enormous grin and fell asleep still smiling, and died over the next two hours, still peaceful and very calm.

Pam was caring for her mother in a remote village, in the family home, which was old fashioned and by her standards poorly equipped. It was not easy for her to manage the washing and general cleaning for the old lady. Her own family lived seven miles away, and she was trying to maintain her own home as well. Her mother was apparently deeply unconscious following a stroke, and it seemed that she could stay like that forever.

Pam, following the advice of some of her mother's older

friends, sat with her for a while and then took her hands and told her: 'You have been a wonderful, Mum. We all love you so much and we will miss you. But we will be all right. We will manage when you have gone; it is all right to let go now, we will all look after each other. Don't worry about us. Just let go and go peacefully.'

She repeated the words several times, then released her mother's hands and sat stroking her arm. Her mother died that night in her sleep. It may be that some people will find the idea repellent or frightening, but Pam felt great relief, and gratitude that she had been able to give the permission that freed her mother from any pressure to fight on. It may seem quite impossible to many people that anyone can have such control over their death, and perhaps it is coincidence, but a coincidence that appears to happen often, though is rarely discussed.

Most people who work with people who are dying will agree that everyone has more control over their death than is ever realised. Even in hospital it is strange how often death will occur at a significant time. Either when everyone is there, or sometimes when everyone has left, if only for a few moments. Often the family will say that that is how the patient would have preferred to die.

Clare, who had been a widow for many years, had some members of her family by her bedside for twenty-four hours a day. She died in the space of a few minutes when they were all outside, planning a rota of who was to stay and who to leave. Only later, her daughter said that she had always hated an audience, and cherished her privacy, and she believed that Clare would have especially hated the audience at such an intensely private time.

All of these examples are anecdotal. There are hundreds more and many that go unreported. Whether the person does die quickly or not, the act of giving permission to let go is often very therapeutic for the family.

Legally, a doctor (GP) must certify death. However, there is often no requirement to call out the GP until the morning. Asking the GP what they would prefer often leads the way to finding out whether the doctor feels there is anything they can do if called. If a family have known their doctor for many years they may feel that he or she will be a good support. If not, or if, as often happens nowadays, there is a locum doctor on call at night, they may feel a stranger will only intrude. Discussing the situation does not make a contract out of whatever is agreed, and should the family feel differently at the time of death, they can always change their minds. However, a doctor *must* certify the death before the funeral director can take the body away. Unless prior arrangements have been made with the funeral director (which sometimes happens), the family will have to keep the body at home until the doctor has made the certification.

Perhaps this is the place to explain that the certificate of death simply certifies that death has taken place. This permits the body to be removed and can be issued by any doctor on call. The death certificate, which is not the same, is the certification of the *cause* of death, and must be issued by a doctor who knows the patient, and has been in recent contact with him or her.

WHEN SHOULD THE FUNERAL DIRECTOR BE INFORMED?

This leads on to another consideration. Funeral directors' charges vary. It may sound very unfeeling, but if someone can consult one or two funeral directors' services early on in the illness, on behalf of the family, it can give them some time in which to choose the service they prefer, and also to compare prices.

Some funeral directors charge extra for a night callout.

Checking these details is something that can be done by a family member or friend. It is also well to remember that the funeral services can be called at the right time for the family.

This is because most funeral directors come within an hour of being called. Knowing how soon they may come means that the family can prepare to let the dead person go. This is a very painful moment, however ready the family may be. If the timing can be chosen carefully and planned for, it is less traumatic for everyone.

For example, the early-morning school rush may seem very public if the family live on the main school run, and have children who would rather not have their school friends see the car leave the house. Or perhaps someone wants to wait for a family member to come home, or to go to work. Sometimes very early in the morning is a quieter time when there is less traffic. The timing is flexible, and should be chosen to suit the family.

WHAT HELP IS AVAILABLE TOWARDS THE END?

Some local health trusts provide help with nursing care for what seems to be the last few hours. The charity Marie Curie Cancer Care can provide a nurse, in partnership with the local trust, at no charge to the family, for several nights when it becomes hard to cope. (Further information is in the Appendix.) Some hospices provide a hospice-at-home service. Investigating the available help at the beginning means that you have some idea of what you can expect.

Alan and Betty had very little time to make arrangements, and with such a young family they could have had the choice of hospice or hospital admission. They were fortunate in that the local hospice offered an 'on call' palliative care service, and when it became apparent that Alan was not going to live very much longer, a nurse was at hand to go out to the family, if she was needed. Betty called her late one night. Alan was very restless, but there was medication in the home to give him if she felt he needed it. The little girls aged eight and ten were there, quiet and calm and watching closely all that happened. They sat in the bedroom and watched a little television and Alan finally settled.

When Alan suddenly became extremely restless, Betty said to the girls that it was as if Daddy was going on holiday and worried about missing the plane, because that was how he always had been when leaving for a trip abroad. It was a good analogy and one that gave a clear picture to the family. Fortunately there was medication available, which alleviated the problem quickly.

When Alan finally settled after having the medication he sank into a deep sleep, and the nurse and the family settled down to get a little rest. Betty lay in her usual position next to him on the big bed, and the children were next door with their door open.

WHAT HELPS THE CHILDREN?

When Alan's breathing stopped at about three a.m. they all heard the sudden silence and gathered in the bedroom. Betty held the children and they wept bitterly for some time. Then they became calmer and talked about what to do. Betty explained she wanted to wash and shave their daddy so that he was smart when the funeral directors came for him, as he always liked to be smart. The oldest girl asked to help. She and Betty washed and shaved him and then Betty asked the children to find something from the garden for him while she and the nurse changed his pyjamas, as he would have felt a bit embarrassed if they had helped with that service. They collected a torch and went off to look in the garden. They came back with a mixed bunch of leaves and flowers, and placed the flowers on his chest, on top of the sheet.

Having cleared away all the traces of pills, and tidied the room, Betty said she would like a cup of tea, and they all sat around talking and playing very softly his favourite Elvis Presley music. The children then asked if they could show the nurse the holiday photos from the year before, and this they did with huge pleasure, and with a lot of laughter and a few tears. The nurse finally left and the family was alone with Alan. Betty phoned the GP, and after his visit the funeral directors arrived at about seven thirty a.m.

Many months later the children were still very composed about the death of their daddy. They spoke of him often, and with a mixture of tears and laughter but no bad dreams. Betty felt that although they missed him terribly, there would never be the reaction that Alan had so wanted to avert, the experience of which, as a child, had affected his life for so long.

Some children do not want to be around at all and will remove themselves from the scene if they can. They should be allowed to follow their own inclination, always remembering that they may be trying to do what they feel adults want. Small ones are really not able to comprehend the fact that they will never see the dead person again, and may make remarks that seem inappropriate and even cruel. They may seem just curious. Whatever the reaction, they need to be able to work through their emotions at their own pace, without criticism.

Sally was just three when her grandma died, and she woke up in the middle of the night to see what was going on. Her aunts and uncles were all there, and she worked her way into the room where they all were, and clutched the only part of her gran that she could reach, which was her big toe. She was lifted up to see her gran and she inspected her carefully and felt her face very gently and announced that her gran was asleep and she, Sally, was ready to go to sleep as well. (Her interpretation of death was accepted for the moment and the explanations about death were left till a later date. It is important that children realise that death is not a sleep state, as they can become frightened of sleeping, or of seeing others asleep, in case they do not wake up.)

Graham, from Chapter Three, had motor neurone disease, and his wife Babs was only in her late twenties when he died from the disease. He had a huge amount of equipment in his room as he was a large man and hard to move. Their three children were all under eight years of age, and Babs had decided exactly what she wanted to do before he died. When he lapsed into unconsciousness, and it seemed that he would die very soon, she dumped all his equipment in the garage, so the room looked like it had always done. She left a note on the door, banning all callers. She played his favourite music and the children sang and crayoned and played with their toys all afternoon. He did not stir but seemed calm and not at all agitated.

They all had their tea with him, and she put them to bed after they kissed him goodnight and goodbye. Her sister came to be there in case the children woke, and Babs went to bed and lay and talked to him and dozed. He died in his sleep in the early hours and she finally called the doctor in the morning. She felt that last day gave her the strength to cope with all the following problems she encountered, as she finally had her husband back for those last hours.

There are some excellent books to help with the confusing experience of the death of a parent or close relative; some can be found at the end of Chapter One.

IS IT POSSIBLE TO DO THE RIGHT THING FOR EVERYONE?

Sometimes families experience great conflict at the point of death. If there are arguments about the sequence of events, then usually it is best to do nothing for the time being.

For example, there are sometimes differing opinions about when to call the funeral directors. Often one member of the family seems to be going against the tide of feelings, and may refuse to allow the body to be taken away. In this case it is better to wait, to leave the dead person in their bed, in a cool room, until the family are united in their readiness to move on. Initially after someone dies there is often a feeling that this is all unreal, and some people may feel that the person cannot really be dead. They will say they are keeping the body forever. Whatever is said in the heat of the moment, if the body is left for a while, to grow cold and less familiar, realisation dawns, and usually it is possible to remove the body without causing a family argument.

Agnes, who lived doors away from her mother, had cared for her for many years. Her siblings saw their mother only once or twice a year. When she died after a short illness, Patsy was deeply grieved to find that the gathered family wanted to clear the house just moments after the body of her mother was taken away, at six a.m. that morning. The family wanted to be on their way and felt they were helping her by clearing away the home. She wanted time to say goodbye to what was in effect her home too. She had a prolonged depression after it was all over.

Some people feel a need to wash and change the body themselves, and this is perfectly all right, and may be a very comforting action. Some find the whole idea uncomfortable, and prefer to leave this to the funeral directors. It is usual to tidy the bed, and close the person's eyes and their mouth, if it is open, and leave the sheet lightly covering the body but with the face uncovered.

It is also appropriate to tidy up hair and replace teeth etc., but only what feels comfortable to the family.

Sylvia was a very attractive and vivacious person who was always immaculately groomed. After she died, Rita, her much loved partner, who had lived with her for fifteen years, and who had provided most of her care during her illness, refused to call the funeral directors until she had completely repainted Sylvia's toe- and fingernails. She arranged with the funeral directors that she would apply the final makeup to Sylvia and do her hair. She said later that for her that was the significant part of the whole experience, the final service she could perform, and something no one else could have done to Sylvia's satisfaction. She felt it was a lovely way to say her goodbyes.

DO PEOPLE NEED MEDICATION UNTIL THEY DIE?

Most medication for symptom relief at the very end of a life is not terribly complex. Advice can be obtained from any hospice or palliative care team, and is usually fairly rapidly effective. This is another reason to make early contact with the palliative care team, rather than wait until the very end of life, when a crisis may occur, and there is no time to plan care. Anxiety can increase the feeling of pain or discomfort, and it is well to plan for this so that appropriate medication is at hand if it is needed. As we have said there is often a fear that the hospice will give medication that may hasten the death of a person. This is a groundless fear but is still prevalent in some areas.

Most palliative care teams have access to 'syringe drivers' and these have become one of the preferred routes for medication, if swallowing becomes difficult. Syringe drivers offer a means of delivering medication via a small needle just under the skin, attached to a battery-run machine, so the medication is given at a planned frequency, in a calculated dose, which can be altered when necessary. There are also suppositories, and skin patches, which give regular doses of medication. These are a tremendous benefit to everyone concerned in symptom relief, professionals and families alike. It means that there is no fear of injections, which can be more painful on very thin and sensitive skin, and ensures

171

that no one suffers pain at the very end because they cannot swallow medication.

As we said earlier, with any illness there is always someone who will give the last injection, just as there is always someone who gives the last bedpan, the last drink, and even the last kiss. If someone dies soon after any treatment, it does not mean that that was the cause of death. Some medication may increase drowsiness, some may cause mild confusion initially, but the idea of offering medication is to alleviate symptoms, and not to end life.

The question of using morphine often causes anxiety with relatives, and yet it is the medication of choice for many symptoms, and will suit the majority of people. There is no fear of addiction if it is being given for symptom relief. Very large doses of morphine can be given with great effect for severe pain and can be reduced if the pain becomes less severe. Pain is depressing and debilitating, and pain reduces the desire to live, and the ability to find some quality in life. Although the large majority of people with cancer do not experience severe pain, it is part of the myth of cancer that everyone expects to suffer a great deal. Many people do not find physical pain the major problem, and if all their concerns can be dealt with honestly, and they can be reassured, the physical pain is eased.

Similarly small doses of morphine can help breathing problems, and if it is offered is always worth trying. Although one of the side effects may be to suppress the breathing mechanics slightly, a small dose will also reduce the fear and panic that accompanies difficulty in breathing, which makes the breathing more stressed. Once again the best course is to ask the professionals.

If someone is severely depressed, sometimes a short spell of anti-depressants may help to lift the mental attitude. It is also worth seeing if talking with someone can relieve their feelings of helplessness.

And for many people, thinking about the concept that we all have some control over our life and our death can give great comfort to someone who feels they have lost control over almost everything else.

IS THERE A PLACE FOR RELIGION?

If someone has a religious faith, that can be a great comfort, but if they do not, then it can be very irritating to have a sermon preached at such a time. A weak and fragile person may well be unable to put a stop to an enthusiastic religious visitor, and may need support from the family to do so. At all times the welfare of the person who is ill should be the first criterion. After that comes the welfare of the people nearest and dearest, who are most affected by the death. The death of a person is the first stage of the experience of bereavement for those closest, and this beginning can make a great difference to the way they look back on the whole course of the illness in later years.

Over the last few years, there has been much research into the power of thought and prayer. There is some evidence that someone who is being prayed for, or has many people thinking about them, recovers more quickly from surgery or treatment than someone who is not. Whether the patient knows they are being prayed for appears to be irrelevant, nor does it matter to whom the prayers are directed. Since prayer does no harm, and may do some good, and will certainly help the person who is praying, there seems to be no reason to reject the offer of prayer, as long as no one objects.

Chapter Eighteen

Dying in Hospital. And a Choice of Funerals?

Sometimes, at the last moment, a hospital admission becomes inevitable. If the family have talked about the dying and planned for it to happen at home, this is a deep disappointment for them. It is hard to come to terms with the fact that all the planning was in vain. But it is not always possible to time a death in such detail, and for many reasons it may be that the hospital becomes, in the end, the appropriate place for the patient.

Hospitals are not as regimented as they once were, and usually it is possible for the family to spend as long as they wish by the bedside, during the last hours, and after the death has occurred, to do the washing of the body as planned. The very fact that there are people around can be a comfort for the family.

Many hospitals have a chapel of rest where family can visit, and sit quietly if they wish. If someone had planned to be at home, and then because of the sudden admission all plans had to change, it can be very comforting to spend a while sitting there, with the dead person, thinking over the last stages of the illness, in peace.

Barry and Jenny had been married for only ten somewhat

sterile and loveless years, when she developed ovarian cancer. She stayed at home, saying very little, while he continued to bury himself in his work. He was away on business when Jenny was taken to hospital – she suddenly developed an unexpected surgical problem. Unfortunately the doctors were not able to operate to cure her and although she went for surgery, they could only relieve the immediate problem, and close the incision, and treat her symptoms with medication. If Barry had been there, he felt, things might have been different and he was racked with guilt, sure that her family would be blaming him for this rushed admission.

He arrived an hour after she died. He spent a long time in her room, sitting by her bed. When he left he seemed calmer and appeared to have come to terms with the death.

Months later he told Jenny's sister Joan that he had talked to Jenny for an hour. He told her he was sorry, not just for this last missed opportunity but for all the times he had not been there for her. He talked to her silent body as he had never talked to her when she was alive. He felt she had heard him. More important, he felt she understood and forgave him. He wished they had had a better marriage but it was not to be.

His sister-in-law did not really understand, but was able to accept what Barry was trying to say. She realised how guilty he felt, but accepted that her sister had once loved this man, and that they had once been happy together. She knew he would lose touch with the rest of the family and was able to let him go without recrimination, glad that her resentment towards him had lessened.

Usually hospital staff are able to give the relative the time and space to be alone with the body and to come to terms with the death.

Children, too, are now more often allowed in hospital to see the body after death, though if the death takes place in the hospital, many people would rather leave the children's involvement until the body is in the funeral directors' chapel.

Again, many families have a need to wash the body themselves, feeling that they want no strangers to be involved in this last service. Most hospital staff will accommodate this request and may even assist the relatives if they wish.

Washing the body is a custom handed down over many years, and is now a matter of choice. Today it is more usually performed by the funeral directors and there is no pressure on the family to be involved, unless they wish.

Funeral directors also will dress the body and add make-up and hair styling if this is required. However, many families fear the body may look artificial, and will suggest doing it themselves. Coffins are not usually left open now for visitors to pay their respects, as they once were, and so the preparation of the body may be seen as less important.

The main thing is that there is no right or wrong process and the wishes of the next of kin are paramount.

The hospital staff will usually be able to call upon a chaplain or priest if they are asked, or the family can contact their own spiritual leader.

To Summarise

Whether it occurs in hospital or at home, the death of a person is intensely private and there is no right or wrong way to meet it. Whatever makes those people most closely concerned feel better is the right action for them. The most important thing is to be left with no feelings of regret, and of being rushed into something.

This may require thinking about dying in a more detailed way than ever before. Some individuals and some communities find this quite natural and have ceremonies, and specific rites to follow, which can be very comforting.

For people without these traditions, thinking about the

death offers an opportunity to plan an individual service that meets their needs and their beliefs.

Funeral Arrangements

Funeral arrangements need planning as well. Many people have strong views about how, or whether, they want to be buried – if this has not been clearly discussed the decision can cause big arguments. This is why it is a good idea to talk about it before death occurs. Often it is something that has been discussed even before the diagnosis was given, and so everyone is aware of the form of service and type of burial or cremation.

Most people who have a religious faith will have a familiar service, and will prefer to stay with that format. What about the people who do not have a faith, and do not want a religious service?

Legally anyone can deliver a funeral service, and coffins can be environmentally kind, if this is specified and planned. It is possible to be buried in a variety of places – even in one's own garden.

There are some people who do want to be buried in the garden of their own home. This needs to be talked through carefully with someone and a good funeral director can help to make the decision.

See the Appendix for details.

★

Whether or not children go to the funeral is the decision of the remaining parent. Babs, Graham's wife, decided she would take the children to the cremation service, but that the coffin would remain stationary until the chapel was empty. She wanted the children to see and to remember how many people had loved their daddy, and she had photos taken of the youthful groups who turned up in dozens, in battered old motorcars and motorbikes, to pay their respects. There were a lot of tears and a lot of laughter too.

When she received the ashes a few weeks later, she took only the oldest boy, who was then nearly nine, to the memorial service and together they sprinkled the ashes under a tree in the gardens of remembrance. Her son told her that he was surprised that the ashes weren't black and she agreed with him. They were able to talk with detachment about the amount of ashes, as they spread them, and then walk away feeling as if the task had been completed. It was a gentle way to say goodbye.

Grace, in her nineties, kept her husband's ashes on the windowsill until she too died, and they could be buried together.

Jean, in an agony of indecision, ended up with her parents' ashes, as well as her husband's ashes, safely in separate jars in her wardrobe. She was constantly teased by her family about this place of safe keeping!

Funerals are for the comfort of the living and so they should be planned to give the maximum support.

People often find it easier to use the words of someone else to express their own feelings of loss and grief, and their beliefs and hopes for whatever comes after death. These do not have to encompass a religious belief or doctrine. To view some of these sayings and writings, there is a website given below, where you can see a selection and use whatever seems appropriate. I have included a few suggestions that you may like to look up as well.

Never be doubtful about including some writing like this, if you are writing to someone recently bereaved – as long as it reflects the sentiments of the person to whom you send it and not your own. It is often hard to find the words to express your feelings without sounding contrived, or trite. If another person has written something and you can use it to comfort someone else, that can only be good.

See website www.poeticexpressions.co.uk/GRIEF.htm.

'Miss me a lot and let me go'	Author unknown
'If I should Die'	Author unknown
'Death is nothing at all'	Canon Henry Scott-Holland
'Comfort'	Elizabeth Jennings
'When I am dead/Remember Me'	Christina Rossetti
'She is Dead / He is Dead'	David Harkins, 1981
'A Special Bridge'	Emily Matthews
'When I must leave you for a while'	Author unknown
'To those I love'	Islo Paschal Richardson
'Only we who Grieve'	Author unknown

Also read:

'Death' by W Somerset Maugham. This is a short and very moving story about meeting death as an appointment we cannot avoid.

'There is a land of the Living and a land of the Dead, and the bridge is Love, the only survival, the only meaning.' Spoken by Brother Juniper, an excerpt from *The Bridge of San Luis Rey* by Thornton Wilder.

Chapter Nineteen

The Effects of Bereavement

Death is only the end for the one who has died. The people left behind have to continue to adjust to, and accept, a whole new group of changes. The obvious change is, of course, the physical loss of the loved one. Although it has been expected, and probably imagined and rehearsed, it is still a completely new experience. It is hard to believe that all the stress is over. For some people the initial reaction is relief, and the feeling that life can now begin again. This is a normal reaction, but it is often followed later on by the anguish of guilt.

There is also a loss of company because carers, who may have been viewed as intruders at the start of an illness, often became friends and allies. And then their job is finished. Some manage to visit once or twice after the death, but they are usually quickly given another patient on whom to focus, and they have to move on.

Friends sometimes do not know what to say. This is common after any bereavement, but if the death has been expected, it is often easier for friends and acquaintances to accept. They have had a while to get used to the idea. If someone has suffered from mental changes like Alzheimer's disease or confusion, or paranoia, then the loss is more like that of a stranger, or comes as a relief to the overstretched carer, and so the acceptance of the loss of the real person has yet to come.

There is always legal business to clarify. Apart from wills and bills, which are the most obvious immediate problems, there are various other details. A woman may have to change her husband's name from all the utilities and perhaps from other legal documents. In future she must pay the bills and the letters must be addressed to her. Pensions, allowances, telephone bills are only a few. Some women have never managed the finances of the house, and in a state of shock feel very incompetent.

A man also may have to start planning and budgeting in a way that he has never before had to consider. He must deal with cooking, and shopping and household chores, and start to use household objects that he may never have noticed before.

Unmarried couples may have legal aspects to clear, and even if there has been good planning and the dead person has tried to make everything simple, it is still an anxious time of readjustment.

For gay couples there can be many difficulties, not the least being that they may not feel free to mourn openly in a society from which they have felt excluded over many years.

There is also the sense of suddenly feeling very vulnerable. The loss of a close friend, or partner, or child, or sibling, is very much like the loss of a limb, and can result in very similar feelings. Physical weakness, unsteadiness, memory loss, sleeplessness, lack of confidence, feelings of helplessness, panic attacks and anxiety, and fear of what lies ahead are all common emotions after someone close has died. It is important to remember that these initial episodes will pass in time or at least become less frequent.

Sometimes there is an inability to weep, and show any outward signs of mourning. This can be caused by disbelief and shock, and can take a long time to resolve.

Sometimes people think they can hear or see the dead person, perhaps in the house, or in bed at night when they turn over they believe they can sense the person lying next to them. Alan and Betty's children often reported they had seen Daddy in the street, or in a shop, or heard Betty talking to Alan at night. Sometimes they seemed happy about it, and sometimes they became upset, but Betty said she also saw him sometimes, and she thought it just meant that he was missing them, and thinking about them. To friends she admitted that she tried hard to relive the sense of his presence as much as possible, and for the first few months she found it a great comfort.

It is certainly not a sign of mental illness to find comfort in that sort of sensation. Anything that gets someone through those first bleak months is acceptable.

There are many good books written about loss. Elisabeth Kübler-Ross has become well known for her explanation and identification of the stages of loss. It is important to remember that the stages she identifies are flexible and the emotions do not appear in a certain order, nor do they last for a specific time, and indeed can repeat and recur for a very long time. Her books, with others, are listed in Further Reading, at the end of this book.

However, not everyone wants to know the pathology of grief. They simply would like a few helpful words on finding a way through the pain. They are told how long it is normal to grieve by well-meaning friends, as well as a wealth of other misinformation. The process of bereavement is like the course of an illness. It is individual and there are no firm rules. *A Grief Observed* by C S Lewis has also given many people insight, comfort and understanding when bewildered by the range of emotions that affects them.

Initial Feelings of Relief

It is not at all unusual to feel initial relief and gratitude that it is all over. The level of anxiety and the fear of not being able to cope is exhausting as well as managing all the physical work involved in caring for someone at home. It is also quite common in people who have made daily hospital journeys for many weeks, which again is a tremendous stress, not always appreciated until it has been experienced.

However, it is rare that this relief lasts long. It may be difficult to sleep in an empty room and an empty house. Familiar noises, soft breathing or a gentle snore have turned to heartbreaking silence. Rather than lie awake for hours, it is often better to get up and walk around and have a warm drink, and try to think back to happy times, or read a book or listen to the radio.

It is also very common to find it hard to concentrate, and pleasures like reading a book, or watching a play, are just not possible for a while. It is hard to enjoy things alone, which were once shared, and now only emphasise the loneliness.

Lisa, after nursing her husband through a very tragic inherited disease, with all the implications for the rest of the family, felt only relief when he finally died. The relief lasted for several years, while she resumed work as a teacher, redecorated the house, tried to remove the memories. She could grieve properly only when she was finally able to remember him as a well person. They had shared many hobbies: running, dancing, reading and gardening, and she had blotted out the fun in the trauma of his illness. She felt great guilt for forgetting so much. She really started grieving for him only four years after his death. Friends did not understand this, and advised her that she should be over it by then, unable to recognise that she was only just starting to miss him.

Maria's family however (Chapter Sixteen) appeared very

relieved after she died and seemed able to continue their lives, still keeping the memory of her alive and fresh, both the times before and after her illness. Their mourning had begun with the diagnosis.

There is no absolute about feelings. It is quite normal to feel a whole range of emotions. Do not allow guilt to intrude on the process of healing.

David (Chapter Eight), when saying how relieved he was feeling after Lee had died, was amused at the comment of a friend who pointed out that his relief was nothing compared to the relief Lee would have felt, if things had been the other way around. He found the remark a source of great comfort when he began to feel guilty. Lee would have hated the restrictions of nursing an ill person, even her much loved husband. She was not at all an instinctive nurse. Indeed they had agreed that if one of them had to be ill, then at least David was the better carer. He managed to remember the real Lee, with her slight imperfections, rather than an idealised image.

Sometimes taking this stance is a comfort. It is surprising how often a couple will agree among themselves that one would cope better than the other, either as a patient, or a carer, or just living alone. And in effect, if they could not die together at the same time, then perhaps the right one died first.

Tim (Chapter Twelve) was consumed with relief, followed by anger and then guilt at being a survivor after Grace died, leaving him with the children to care for. Reading through Grace's memory book helped him a great deal. He realised that she had hoped that he would be glad for her when it was all over, and that he would keep her memory alive without any regrets. And he remembered her wish that he would be happy again one day.

Coping With Feelings of Guilt and Regret

People feel guilty for many reasons. There is the feeling of never having done enough. Of the times when everything seemed too hard and care was given grudgingly because the carer was tired out. And, too often, the feeling of guilt at being the survivor.

There is also guilt when life begins to be happy again. It can seem wrong to enjoy life when a loved one is not there to join in.

Alan and Betty from Chapters Two, Five and Seventeen had two children of ten and eight. After he died Betty found life very hard and said she really felt she would never be happy again. One day she and the children started laughing at something on television and her eldest daughter stopped and said, 'It doesn't seem right for us to be laughing and Daddy can't join in.'

The younger girl replied, 'Daddy was always the first one to laugh and he wouldn't recognise us now.'

Betty thought a lot about this, and remembered the laughter they had shared, and realised how much the children missed Alan's sense of fun. She decided to make changes that day, and she did, though it was not always easy. For her this was the first step on the slow road to recovery: the recognition that she could still laugh without being disloyal to her dead husband.

Most people, if asked, would agree that they want to be remembered without feelings of negativity and guilt. Most people would like to feel they will be remembered with laughter and pleasure when they are dead.

Moreover, if asked the question 'What do you think your husband/wife/child/parent might say if they were here now? Would they say you should have done more/less/differently?' most people would agree that they did all they could at the time, and in those circumstances. If the relationship has deteriorated, it is important to remember how it once was, before the illness ravaged the emotions, and when they supported each other wholeheartedly, and with love.

Everyone has their own way of coping and feelings like guilt form a part of the pattern. But guilt is negative and does not promote healing.

Regrets are easier to manage. Everyone has regrets, because it is impossible to live through such an experience with textbook perfection. Everyone can do only their best, and their best may never seem good enough.

The most painful regrets are often associated with having not said enough, rather than not done enough.

Margaret and John (Chapter Thirteen) had not been happy for a long time, and after he died she began to wish they had been able to make some small link before his death. She wrote a letter to him, telling him how she felt, and saying that she would try to look back with generosity on their life together. It was quite a formal letter, but she felt better afterwards. She was not quite sure of what to do with it, as he was long since buried, so she kept it for a while. One day she burned it in the garden, and watched the ashes disintegrate, and with them allowed the guilt and regrets to leave her.

If there has been no opportunity to talk freely while someone is ill, or if there has not been openness in the relationship before the illness, it is hard to change a pattern of behaviour in times of extreme stress. Sometimes there is a longing for a few spontaneous words like 'I love you.' If they have not been freely said for many years, it is a hard request to make when someone is especially vulnerable.

Sometimes there is only a chance to speak after the death. Mark's father (Chapter Five) was never able to talk to either his son or his wife, and seemed to deal with the whole experience by denying it was happening. After his wife died he spent two hours in her room, alone with her body, talking continuously. No one could hear what was said, but he seemed very calm when he left her room, and later asked Mark if he had anything to say to his mother, before the funeral directors came. Mark sat with her for a while, and appeared to be deep in thought, but said nothing aloud. He kept his emotions tightly under control, as he had always done. Fortunately his teacher continued the support he had given, even after Mark left his school.

Many people put a note in the coffin and this can be a very satisfying way to say what is needed to end an experience. Some people plant a tree or a rose as a way of leaving the past behind, but remembering the person with affection.

Losing Contacts After Death

Many people after a long illness at home feel very alone after the professionals involved leave the house. They cannot imagine life without all the interruptions. These strangers have become friends, and they provided a structure for the day. When all the aids and equipment have gone, the house seems very bare. It can be hard to remember a life before the illness. Often friends have gradually come less frequently, and the bonds have weakened and there is no one around who appears to understand the feelings of the carer.

Friends also have seen the changes in the patient, and often make inappropriate comments based on how they interpret the situation. They may assume that there is great relief that the experience is at an end, or they may criticise actions of professionals, or they may offer advice that is quite unrealistic. Or else they simply do not know what to say and keep away. The bereaved person may become the one who has to make the first move, and also guide the friends in their responses.

There are so many different ways of approaching all

these reactions. Honesty is usually the best approach, but may result in a lost friendship, with saying something like: 'I wish you wouldn't criticise so and so/offer so many ideas/assume that I am happy this is all over/think I should have done things differently/because it makes me feel so inadequate/because it's so hurtful/I would rather not talk about meeting someone else right now – I simply can't begin to think about that/I do appreciate seeing you today – it makes me feel as if I am still part of life. I have missed the contact with old friends.'

Sadly there will always be some people who simply look the other way when faced with someone in deep grief. It is hurtful but it is a fact. There may come a time when they will make a fresh approach, but there is no point in becoming obsessed with their inadequacies. It is better to look for the friends who can help.

See the end of this book for telephone numbers for getting help with your bereavement.

Chapter Twenty

Supporting a Friend. What to Say, and What Not to Say

Society today is not used to saying nothing. We like to offer advice. But sometimes there is nothing to say that can give comfort. Sometimes silence is the most comforting support. Just sitting silently and responding if required. It is good to have someone close enough to understand, but if there is no one then some of the charities are very helpful in sending a visitor around to provide what is needed emotionally. There need be no shame in asking for help, any more than in calling for the doctor to bandage a wound.

People who have not experienced loss themselves often assume reactions and, as we have said, suggest a reasonable time for grieving. Two years seem to be an accepted time – then the grief should have healed, they say.

This can only be a very arbitrary and uninformed view. Each loss is individual and cannot be measured. Some people would say that no one ever recovers from a death, but they learn to live with the loss and even to be happy again.

Loss of a loved person is affected by someone's age, personal history, length and degree of illness, length and depth of relationship, the amount of support available, and many other factors. The assumption that everything can be quantified and prescribed is nonsense.

What Helps?

Silence helps, as was said previously. Undemanding companions can be very supportive if they are aware and the silence is supportive and the companion does not stay for hours and hours.

Listening helps. Sometimes the only way to absorb and realise the loss is for the person who has been bereaved to talk about it, to go over and over what has happened, how it happened, who said what and when. They go over the whole story over and over again, until they can assimilate the event. This happens with any loss, and virtually any great emotional shock. If you have ever lost your house keys or had something stolen from you, or experienced a severe shock, you may remember how many times you needed to tell your story. A good listener is a tremendous asset, and anyone who is aware of this can be a great support at a time of tragedy.

Inviting someone round for a quick informal cup of tea is helpful, if a specific time is given. Often the bereaved person finds it hard to leave the house at first, though some people may find it hard to stay *in* the house. Either way, an invitation for an informal chat can show support and friendship and be a great comfort.

Short visits are also better than long ones. Many people find grief exhausting. If a visitor is in doubt about when to leave, asking a person to say when they are tired is a way of offering options. It may be too hard to say 'Please go now, I've had enough' but if asked a direct question it is possible to agree, 'Yes, I am tired' without fearing that the visitor will take offence and not come again.

There is no need to deluge anyone with flowers, and

initially after any bereavement most people have rooms full of blooms. It is a few weeks before the visits tail off and the flowers with them. That is when a few flowers bring pleasure and appreciation. Men are rarely given flowers, and yet many men very much appreciate them.

As we have said, listening helps. It also helps if the listener can recall memories of the dead person. Visitors often feel embarrassed in case they cause tears, and initially, of course, they will do. But talking helps to make the loss a reality and tears can be very healing. As time goes by the tears will become fewer, simply as someone learns to control them.

Recounting memories, especially occasions that were very happy or funny, are tremendously comforting, and add to the feeling that to a degree other people share the loss. Chris's mother (Chapter Four) was deeply touched when she was told by a neighbour that he and his family had missed hearing Chris singing in the shower when he first left home to work in the city. She had never realised how the sound carried, and was then able to talk freely to her about the days when he was small, and playing in the garden. They spoke together of his schooldays, of planning his career, and how she missed him when he finally flew the nest.

Paul's son (Chapter Fourteen) was able to reduce the family to tears and laughter by saying 'open wide' whenever he felt like being the centre of attention, for many months after Paul had died. All the children liked to talk about the times when he was alive, and the sort of things they did together as a family.

Asking questions is fine too: 'How did you first meet?' 'I had no idea that you were such keen walkers.' 'Do you remember when we moved in and...came over with some tea for us?'

Anyone who has known someone for even a short time has a personal view of them and a relevant memory to share.

What Does Not Help?

As we have seen, avoiding someone is not helpful, and in fact adds considerably to the grief. Even if no word is spoken, and a hug or handshake is all that is offered, that can be very comforting.

Anything that may appear to minimise the loss is unhelpful. This includes remarks like: 'You're young and you're bound to meet someone else.' 'Fortunately you've got the children.' 'He/she has gone to a better place.' 'He's better out of it all.' 'You were lucky to have had such a happy marriage/good relationship.'

Any of these remarks may be made by the person who has suffered the loss, but not by someone who is trying to comfort them.

When the marriage has been obviously unhappy, or when the carer has complained a lot about the hard work, it is still not helpful to assume that they will feel relief after death. Assume nothing and simply acknowledge the feelings he or she demonstrates. It is not a question of being insincere, if someone has been bereaved – it is not for anyone else to judge how they may be feeling.

Sharing experiences of death is rarely helpful either. A person recently bereaved can think only about their own loss, and cannot be expected to listen and comfort another person reliving their grief. Knowing they share an experience is enough, without hearing all the details.

Telling lots of jokes, and trying to bring laughter is not helpful either. Some people are spontaneously and incorrigibly funny, but they are rare. If something occurs that is humorous, then that is a bonus, but thinking up funny things is not usually helpful, especially when it is obviously a contrived humour not naturally there.

Certainly recalling amusing or affectionate memories can bring a mix of tears and laughter, and that is also a comfort as was said earlier in this chapter. A visitor who sheds a few tears with the bereaved person can be a comfort, but someone who is so upset that they require comforting, and who weeps loud and long, is a liability.

Anniversaries

Anniversaries are not only the traditional occasions like Christmas and birthdays. After someone dies there is a whole new range of anniversaries, which can be seen as the first and last anniversaries. The dates of the first anniversary can be the appearance of the first symptoms, the first visit to hospital, or the day of the diagnosis, or the missed holidays. The last anniversaries may be the last birthday, the last day out, the last meal, the last laugh with friends or family.

In many ways life starts afresh from the date of death, almost like a child beginning a new life. But beyond the starting date is another whole world, and it can be relived relentlessly for the first year at least.

For many people the first traditional public anniversaries are the most difficult to acknowledge, because they are often public celebrations, which are dreaded beforehand, and give relief when they are over. There can also be almost a slight easing of pain when the first year is over. The first Christmas, the first birthday, the first spring, the first public holiday are all painful reminders of what used to be. Nothing really helps, and this is a stage that everyone has to go through, when the emotions are raw and extreme.

The pain is different as anniversaries continue to arrive. Often the second and third years are sad because there is the realisation that the loss is permanent, and with this realisation is the fear of memories beginning to fade, and then ultimately forgetting, and losing the essence of this much loved person.

Time really is the only healer, and even so perhaps healing

is too much to ask for. Perhaps all anyone will ever do is learn to live with the loss.

Inappropriate Reactions

Sometimes people are puzzled by what they see as strange and inappropriate reactions in the person who has been left. We all accept and to an extent understand the person who breaks their heart over the death of a pet, and yet appeared stoical over the loss of a partner or parent a while before. We imagine they are transferring their grief to a more manageable level. Often it is easier to cry over a sentimental film, or a sad item in the news, than over the death of someone much loved. This is quite normal and helps to reduce the burden of sadness that has built up internally.

Similarly, a history of several losses can accumulate over time, and in old age a woman can appear to weep inappropriately for a friend, when in fact they are also grieving for the loss of a long-dead sibling or parent. They are grieving for long-past sadness and loss, or even for their own approaching age and loss of faculties.

It is not uncommon to see an extreme public response to the death of a public figure, and in a way this may also be a way of dealing with buried personal losses over many years. The extreme reaction is a more recent phenomenon, but it has to be accepted as perhaps helpful in many ways for some people.

As time goes by, different losses come into focus. For both young and old people the loss of touch and intimacy is very hard to bear. Widows often say, after years of widowhood, that they still miss holding someone's hand, or feeling someone's arm around them. And at any age, the loss of sexual intimacy can be very hard to bear.

It is true that sometimes antidepressants can help for a short time in some cases. Some homeopathic remedies are also useful. Most medication has a numbing effect, and to recover from bereavement most authorities agree one has to experience the pain, and grow through it. It helps to have a sympathetic GP with whom to talk over the feelings and who will suggest medication if it seems likely to be helpful.

Clearing Away Belongings

For some people, clearing away all the personal effects of the dead person is helpful. Others may hold onto those items for a long time, and some even sleep with a familiar coat or jacket. It is an individual choice and cannot be hurried or managed by anyone else. Usually, the time comes when it is bearable to allow those memories to go, and that is another stage of the recovery process.

To be pushed and bullied into parting with them is neither helpful nor kind.

Similarly, moving house is not an easy choice, even when the plans have been made and agreed on, long before the death.

Sometimes the person left behind is very ready to leave the house. Nicholas, very soon after Rose died (Chapter Sixteen) sold the house and moved to a very different environment. He settled well but his children and he had little contact after that, not just because he had left the family home.

Maria's family (also Chapter Sixteen) kept the house very much as she had left it and also kept all her clothes for nearly a year, giving them away over time, to specific charities or friends.

After Jeanette had died, Edward (Chapter Sixteen) was very quick to change the entire kitchen and redo it to his taste as he said he would be doing a lot of the cooking in the future. The girls joined in, and they were so pleased with the result that they continued over the whole house.

It seemed to be a therapeutic exercise for the whole family, but also an expensive one, and not always possible because of the cost.

Some people give away clothes and get pleasure from the idea that they might see someone wearing familiar clothes that they no longer need. For others this is too painful, and they will travel a distance to donate clothing for charity, in an area where they will not be likely to see someone else wearing familiar items.

Everyone is different, so there is no right or wrong response, as long as it feels right to those most closely concerned. Certainly some people seem never to recover from the loss of a loved one, and after many years together it is easy to understand why recovery is slow, and perhaps impossible.

Of course there are some people who become severely depressed and the grief is too great a burden for them. The kind of pathological grief personified in the extreme by Queen Victoria needs to be addressed, and can often be treated with some success by a psychiatrist, or similar specialist. The source for this help is the GP – a good GP will be aware of the possibility of this problem and hopefully will be observing the patient at regular intervals.

Chapter Twenty-one

Starting a New Life Alone

Sometimes the hardest part of recovery is getting out and about, without the other person. There are some similar reactions to look out for in both sexes, but also quite different ones. For example, in general, a man who is on his own is seen as being easier to accommodate in a social environment than a single woman, and therefore men are often invited out more frequently than women. However, both men and women, when left on their own, can lapse into a despondent attitude and become unkempt and scruffy, resulting in social exclusion that only makes the situation worse for them.

Some people make a desperate attempt to fill their loneliness by rushing into new relationships too early, which can result in personal hurt and disappointment for them, as well as other people less closely involved like families and friends. Women and men do this: they are looking for an identical replacement for their loss, almost a balm for the pain they are experiencing. Some of these relationships thrive, but many do fall apart fairly quickly.

It is sometimes said that men are better able to move on and start again without carrying a lot of regrets about the past, and without trying to replicate the dead partner. This may be true in some circumstances, but it is impossible to generalise, as everyone has their own response and individual reaction.

Both sexes often find the experience of socialising very difficult after the death of a partner. Men can go to pubs but often find the loneliness accentuated, particularly if this is a new activity. Older people may find it hard because they do not have the experience of mixing socially in clubs and places where younger folk may feel quite at home.

Almost everyone has a view of what is hard and what is manageable. The question is how to meet the new position with optimism and enjoyment.

There has been a huge increase in singles clubs, but people who have been fairly recently bereaved may not welcome this idea. This is not to say that they do not have their place for some people. Often, after a while, younger people will look at the services offered by these clubs as a way of getting back into a social life, as much as a way of seeking a new relationship. It is hard at any age to find oneself alone in a society that is directed to a large extent at couples. Even going on holiday can be hard when generally all the prices quoted are for couples and, in fact, single bookings can often incur penalties. When friends make attempts at matchmaking the results can be embarrassing, and can exaggerate the feelings of failure and isolation.

Joining a walking club, a gardening club, a bridge club or special interest club is often the best way to meet other people with similar interests. The environment in this type of club is less pressured, and it is easier to integrate slowly, and get to know people as a single person.

Often the best attitude is to get involved in anything that seems interesting, so that you can meet as many new friends as you can manage, without feeling pressured. Nothing can replace the lost relationship, and in fact sometimes for a time a new interest or activity can almost increase the sense of loss, and of losing the person, because the new interest cannot be shared, as once it would have been. But this emotion will pass, and a new concern can fill some of the emptiness in the meantime.

A supportive family is a great blessing, but the temptation to involve one's life wholly with family can also be restricting. It helps to reach out for new friends and activities, so that the family do not have to feel responsibility for you, nor you for them.

It also helps to have a structure to the day. Caring for someone for any length of time means the carer has a job, a structure to the day, since they have to perform certain tasks at certain times. This structure goes when they are finally left alone, and it is very hard to replace it. Household chores, cooking and doing the garden, cease to be rewarding when there is no one there to comment on the result, or to offer a suggestion, or to praise the industriousness of the worker. Even making tea for one has the effect of reducing the desire for tea, let alone cooking a meal. Any activity that can provide a structure for the day is good.

Kapila, a wonderful cook, started to share meals with her neighbour. They took it in turns to cook for each other, which must have made a great difference to both of them, providing both with delicious meals and company, especially in the winter evenings.

Although only the person concerned can help themselves in this way, friends can help a little by non-pressured invitations. It may take many months of apathy and reluctance before starting a new interest or gaining the commitment to attend a course or a hobby. The idea may not be viewed with any measure of enthusiasm. But the time will come. Going out alone, and coming into an empty house can be painful, and is a continual reminder of how life has changed, but it gets more manageable with practice.

The difficulties are different with different age groups. People married for many years find it hard to make the adjustment to a single state. Young people with families may also find it hard financially and practically, to get into a very different routine. The surviving partner of a gay couple may be very isolated at work, because colleagues do not realise the significant loss of an unacknowledged relationship, and therefore the remaining partner can never talk about the lost love. Anyone suddenly losing a partner feels like the 'odd one out' because wherever they are there is often a spare seat at the table and the sense of something missing. Whatever the position, if friends are supportive and patient and continue to call, they will be a great help.

New Relationships

There is no right time for a new relationship. As said earlier on, sometimes after a very happy marriage someone will be anxious to replace the lost love as quickly as possible. This can result in some pain for several people, as emotions are sometimes very haphazard for a long time after a loss. It is also not uncommon for someone to feel a sudden and passionate attachment to someone who has been especially kind and supportive to them over the period when their loved one was ill, or immediately afterwards.

Ann, a young woman when her husband died, fell into several passionate and short-lived relationships in the year after his death. Fortunately she kept them to herself, so that when she became more emotionally stable, and understood that she could not replace her husband in that way, she did not have to listen to the judgements of her friends and relatives. She was able to accept and not feel too guilty about her experiences, as no one else had been aware of what she regarded as her 'lapses'. She had had a very happy marriage and she believed that her husband would have understood very well her need for physical affection after his death.

As we have said earlier there will be some people who

will never be able to begin a new life that has any real value for them.

Tom was an old man who lost his wife and then his only daughter within a year. Wrapped up in his grief he spent each Thursday walking in the hospice gardens remembering the Thursday when his dear wife died. The hospice were able to accommodate this need of his to be near where she died, by finding the odd job he could do for them while he was there. But the intensive care unit, in the hospital where his daughter died after a road accident, were not able to give him time and company each weekend, when he sat quietly outside in the corridor. He often brought cake or biscuits for the staff, all of whom felt very sad for him, but really were not able to give him the help he needed. They finally managed to wean him away from the unit, after he arrived with some of his daughter's clothes, and the sister persuaded him to take them to a charity shop. There he found a kindly soul with whom to chat, and he spent a lot of time there, until he himself died a year or so later.

Bereavement is an individual experience with some aspects common to everyone, and some unique to each person. Sometimes a friend or relative is worried that the whole process is taking too long, or perhaps the person seems to be unable to move on emotionally after a very long time, at least several years. In this case it is best to talk openly with sensitivity about your concerns to that person, without giving the impression that they are maximising their grief. You could suggest seeing a bereavement counsellor, or their doctor, if they will agree. There often comes a stage when, however painful the loss, they no longer want to carry the pain around with them, and will think about asking for help. Sometimes it takes an outsider who cares about them to identify a state of depression, which can be treated.

At some point all of us will experience the loss of someone we love. Trying to avoid love is a lonely way to try and avoid the pain. Learning to accept and work through the loss is part of living that cannot be avoided. Helping another person at such a time is a privilege for the helper and also a learning experience that we may need ourselves one day. It is not only a chance to give, but also a chance to receive and gain valuable insight. To ignore the opportunity is to lose a valuable experience.

We are at the end of this book. Many people have contributed to the ideas here. All of them lived and died in their own unique fashion. The people who loved them have had to move on. All of us who knew them learned from them and remember them with gratitude, with sadness, with admiration and often with humour. Knowing them has enriched our lives.

Richard Reoch in his book *Dying Well* wrote:

'What you give to others is not merely what you possess; what you leave to others is not solely what you have accomplished. At every moment in your life and in the period of your dying you shape the future of others. You do this in many ways, but the most powerful and the most persuasive is the impact that you make upon other people's understanding of themselves and of their underlying attitudes to life. One of the greatest legacies you can leave them is the impact of your own preparation for death, your own understanding of it and the manner of your dying.'

Appendix

Support for Carers

BEFRIENDING NETWORK

Can put you in touch with similar networks nationally as well as providing local volunteer support in the north and west London.

Tel 020 7689 2443
Web www.befriending.net

CARERS UK

Helpline 0808 808 7777, only part time in the week. They can also give information on help for young carers who are often deeply involved when a parent is ill.

Tel 020 7490 8818
Web www.carersonline.org.uk

THE PRINCESS ROYAL TRUST FOR CARERS

Can also give information on services available for carers and for young carers.

Tel 020 7480 7788

General Help, Practical and Financial

BENEFITS ENQUIRY LINE

Confidential advice on all the benefits available, and how to claim them, and how to fill in the forms in some cases.

Helpline 0800 882200
Web www.dss.gov.uk

BRITISH RED CROSS

Tel 020 7235 5454
Web www.redcross.org.uk

Or call your local branch for practical help like loans of certain equipment and transport.

DISABLED LIVING FOUNDATION

Provides advice and information on equipment of all types by phone or letter or email. They also have a demonstration centre.

Helpline 0845 130 9177
Web www.dif.org.uk

NHSDirect

Provides a twenty-four-hour helpline for advice on many health issues and information on medical conditions and health services and support groups in your area.

Helpline 0845 4647
Web www.nhsdirect.nhs.uk

The Rosetta Life Project

As mentioned in Chapter Twelve

Tel 020 7520 8270
Email lucinda.jarrett@rosettalife.org

Samaritans

They provide a listening ear but do not offer advice. Look in your local telephone directory.

Care and Services for People With Cancer

The Hospice Information Service

This service gives information about local hospice services in your area as well as being an international resource for professionals and for the public.

Tel 0870 903 3903

Marie Curie Cancer Care

The charity is partly funded by local services, and the nurses are locally employed so the district nurse or the GP are the people to contact. The assessment for the need of a Marie Curie nurse is made by the district nurse. They work for a short period of time when the need is greatest, and they usually work a shift of never fewer than nine hours. For this reason they are of tremendous help overnight in enabling the carer to enjoy a much needed sleep.

Tel 020 7599 7777 for information about the service in your area

Breast Cancer Care

Helpline 0808 800 6000
Web www.breastcancercare.org.uk

Cancer Black Care

Offers help specifically for minority groups affected by cancer, and also has a befriending programme.

Helpline 020 7249 1097

Cancer Research UK

Helpline 0800 226237
Cancer information nurses 020 7061 8355
Web www.cancerresearchuk.org and www. cancerhelp.org.uk

Offers information and leaflets.

CANCERBACUP

Provides wide support for people affected by the disease including specific cancers and their treatments. They also have a service linked to an interpreter called Cancer in Your Language.

Helpline 0808 800 1234
Web www.cancerbacup.org.uk

MACMILLAN CANCERLINE

Provides a service and information for people with the disease, and their families.

Helpline 0808 808 2020
Web www.macmillan.org.uk

NATIONAL CANCER ALLIANCE

Tel 01865 793566

BRISTOL CANCER HELP CENTRE

Works with medical treatment to offer emotional, physical and spiritual care to the whole family.

Helpline 0845 1232310
Web www.bristolcancerhelp.org

Exit

17 Hart Street, Edinburgh EH1 3RN
Tel 0131 556 4404, fax 0131 557 4403
Email exit@euthanasia.cc

Exit supports voluntary euthanasia and offers discussion and advice on this subject. They will also offer advice on living wills and the problems associated with them.

Care and Services for Non-cancer Illness and Disease

Look in your local telephone directory for local and national support groups.

G-Text

This is a directory of UK self-help groups, now in its tenth edition. There is a charge for the directory.

> **Tel** 01253 402237
> **Web** www.ukselfhelp.info

Voluntary Agencies Directory

This can be found in the local library.

Leonard Cheshire Care

Provides care and support for disabled people as well as for people with learning disabilities all over the UK.

> **Tel** 020 7802 8200 for information, or look in your local directory

Sue Ryder Care

Has eighteen centres in Britain for people with many different diseases and disabilities.

> **Tel** 020 7400 0440 for information or look in your local directory

Mobility

People can apply for financial help with vehicles if they have a disabling illness. So ask for information through your local services or doctor.

Motability

If you are having difficulty driving your car, or if you are having to depend on friends and family for help, it is worth contacting the helpline if only to clarify your situation. Motability offers advice and helps with the application forms you may require. Talk to your occupational therapist.

> **Helpline** 0845 456 4566
> **Web** www.motability.co.uk

Queen Elizabeth Foundation Mobility Centre

The centre can assess for disability and suggest adaptations to current vehicles for anyone who can get to their centre. There is a charge for this detailed assessment. For people with motor neurone disease they have a *special vehicle loan service, which can be long term or short term, and which has to be accessed through the Motor Neurone Disease Association regional care advisors.*

> **Tel** 020 8770 1151
> **Web** www.quefd.org/mobilitycentre

Medication – Information

British National Formulary describes the interaction of drugs and their side effects. Can be bought outright from most bookshops, ISBN 0-85369-380-3. Specific information can be obtained from

Pain Relief – Information

The Pain Society, 21 Portland Place, London W1B 1PY
Email info@painsociety.org

If you are unable to get help with your pain locally through the services available to you, the Pain Society can give addresses of pain clinics in the UK.

The Pain Relief Foundation Clinical Sciences Centre

University Hospital, Aintree, Liverpool L9 7AL
Web www.painrelieffoundation.org.uk

Send a 50p sae and specify the kind of pain and the health problem.

Complementary Therapies

HOMEOPATHY
Homeopaths in your area can be found from:

The Register of Homeopaths
Tel 0845 4506611
Fax 0845 4506622
Email info@homeopathy-soh.org

Or look in your local directory or take personal recommendation.

Holidays

St Christopher's Hospice has an excellent fact sheet on holidays.

Tel 0208 778 9252

All the relevant charities will have some information about holidays or respite care. Telephone them or ask someone who has the time to look it up on the internet for you. This is something that is easy to do and a way of helping without being inconvenienced.

Funerals

NATURAL DEATH CENTRE

Offers comprehensive information on all aspects of death and funeral options.

Tel 0871 2882098
Web www.naturaldeath.org.uk

Some people have a desire to have a *green funeral* and there is an increasing interest in biodegradable coffins. Information about these is from:

GREENFIELD COFFINS LTD

Unit 6–7 Lakes Road, Braintree, Essex CM7 3SS
Tel 01440 788886
Fax 01440 788877
Email sales@greenfieldcoffins.com

GREEN ENDINGS FUNERALS LTD

Tel 020 7424 0345
Web www.greenendings.co.uk

What to do After a Death is a free leaflet from the DSS and is available from post offices.

Bereavement

CHILD BEREAVEMENT NETWORK

Provides information and help for bereaved children and the people who care for them as well as other caregivers.

Tel 020 7843 6309
Web www.nob.org.uk/cbn!directory

CRUSE BEREAVEMENT CARE

126 Sheen Road, Richmond TW9 1VR

Offers support to people as well as information and advice.

Helpline 0870 167 1677, or send a sae for leaflets and publications.

JEWISH BEREAVEMENT COUNSELLING SERVICE

Offers help to all family members.

Tel 020 8385 1874
Web www.jvisit.org.uk/jbcs
Email jbcs@jvisit.org.uk

LESBIAN AND GAY BEREAVEMENT PROJECT

c/o The Healthy Gay Living Centre, 40 Borough
High Street, London SE1 1XW
Tel 020 7403 5969

Provides help for the bereaved person and also to family and
friends. It also gives advice on wills for same sex partners.

WINSTON'S WISH

The Clara Burgess Centre, Bayshill Road,
Cheltenham GL50 3AW
Tel 01242 515157
Email info@winstonswish.org.uk
Web www.winstonswish.org.uk

Supports young people who have experienced death of a
close family member. They provide help, advice, resources
and publications.

★

This is not a comprehensive list. If you ask, all of these
contacts will be able to put you in touch with other services
available.

Further Reading

BOOKS FOR ADULTS ABOUT DIFFERENT ASPECTS OF CARING,
DEATH, AND BEREAVEMENT

A Grief Observed, C S Lewis, Faber & Faber, ISBN 0-571-06624-
0. Lewis's insight into his own grief after his wife died.
Dying Well, Richard Reoch, Gaia Books, ISBN 1-85675-019-1.
Have the Men Had Enough?, Margaret Forster, Penguin, ISBN
0-140-12769-0.

How to Survive Bereavement, Andrea Kon, Hodder & Stoughton, ISBN 0-340-78624-8.

I Don't Know What to Say, Robert Buckman, Macmillan, ISBN 0-333-54035-2.

Living with Death and Dying, Elisabeth Kübler-Ross, Collier Books, ISBN 0-02-086490-6.

The Natural Death Handbook, Stephanie Wienrich and Josefine Speyer, ISBN 1-8441322-6-9.

On Children and Death, Elisabeth Kübler-Ross, Collier Books, ISBN 0-02-076670.

On Death and Dying, Elisabeth Kübler-Ross, Routledge, ISBN 0-41504-015-9.

Remind Me Who I Am Again, Linda Grant, Granta, ISBN 1-86207-171-3. This is a compassionate and honest book about the experiences of caring for a relative with MID or Multi-Infarct Dementia, which is sometimes confused with Alzheimer's disease.

The Selfish Pig's Guide to Caring, Hugh Marriott, Polperro Heritage Press, ISBN 0-9544233-1-3. The title speaks for itself and is a humorous and very insightful way of looking at the whole business of becoming a carer.

Staying Alive – A family memoir, Janet Reibstein, Bloomsbury, ISBN 0-7475-6470-1. About a family legacy of breast cancer.

Tuesdays With Morrie, Mitch Albom, Doubleday (New York), ISBN 0-385-48451-8. The story of Mitch's tutor who died of motor neurone disease and how he responded to the illness.

When the Crying's Done, Jeannette Kupfermann, Robson Books, ISBN 0-86051904-X. A widow's account.

BOOKS FOR CHILDREN

Am I Still a Sister?, Alicia M Sims, Gilgal Publications, ISBN 0-9618995-0-6. Caring for the dying at home.

Badger's Parting Gifts, Susan Varley, Collins Picture Lions, ISBN 0-00-6643175-5.

Beginnings and Endings with Lifetimes in Between, Bryan Mellonie and Robert Ingpen, Dragon World, ISBN 1-85028-038-X.

The Fall of Freddie the Leaf, Leo Buscaglia Slack, ISBN 0-8050-1064-5.

Goodbye Mog, Judith Kerr, Collins, ISBN 0-00-714969-7.

Gran's Grave, Wendy Green, Lion Press, ISBN 0-7459-1556-6.

How it Feels When a Parent Dies, Jill Krementz, Gollancz, ISBN 0-575-05183-3.

Name all the Animals, Alison Smith, Scribner (New York), ISBN 0-743-25522-4.

The Tenth Good Thing About Barney, Judith Viorst, Aladdin Paperbacks, ISBN 0-689-71203-0.

Waterbugs and Dragonflies, Doris Stickney Mowbray, ISBN 0-264-66904-5.

When Uncle Bob Died, Althea Dinosaur Publications, ISBN 0-85122-727-9.

BOOKS FOR ADULTS TO WORK THROUGH WITH CHILDREN

There are books for children to write in and record feelings and fears around the death of a parent or sibling. These can be of great benefit but require a sensitive approach and the child must want to take part in the process.

When Someone Very Special Dies, Marge Heegaard, Woodland Press, ISBN 0-9620502-0-2.

CPSIA information can be obtained at www.ICGtesting.com
Printed in the USA
LVOW12s2145111113

360944LV00018B/289/P